Aussie Women Don't Fear Fat

A Practical Aussie Path to a Lighter Life

JACINTA PLAZZER

BOOKS
WITH HEART
by Jacinta

Books with Heart by Jacinta Publishing

NATIONAL
LIBRARY OF AUSTRALIA

Legal Deposit:

A copy of this publication has been deposited with the **National Library of Australia** in accordance with the *Copyright Act 1968*.

ISBN: 978-0-6487554-1-8

e-ISBN 978-0-6487554-2-5

Edited and designed in Australia.

Dedicated to Heidi and Freya.

Live Fearlessly.

Later I will know myself more clearly.

Rosemary Dobson

Contents

APPENDICES

Introduction

It has been 20 years since Mireille Guiliano told the world, in her now-iconic book, that *French Women Don't Get Fat*. Soon after, Naomi Moriyama and William Doyle informed us that *Japanese Women Don't Get Old or Fat*, and suddenly the world was intrigued all over again.

The first book created a global curiosity, almost a longing.

I embraced my inner Frenchwoman. Later, my inner Japanese. I bought the small bowls, the chopsticks, the tiny plates and the wabi-sabi perfectly imperfect ceramics. I walked to the shops, slowed down my meals, ate with more "awareness" and savoured smaller portions. For a while, it all felt charming... exotic... clever.

Both cultures do food beautifully, from the French infusion of ritual, elegance and an enviable calm around eating, to the Japanese balance, lightness and the simple pleasure of stopping at eighty per cent full. In each place, food is more than fuel; it is ritual, beauty and art.

Meanwhile, most Australian women grew up nowhere near Paris or Tokyo.

We did not grow up with three-hour lunches, tiny pastries, elegant restraint, or the social pressure to appear perfectly composed at every meal. We did not grow up in a world where eating slowly was expected, where sharing small plates was standard, or where "listening to your body" was a daily practice rather than something many of us do not truly learn until our forties.

We grew up in Australia, the land of BBQs, beach days, brunches, generous servings, pavlova, wine o'clock, beer o'clock and the national motto, "Help yourself, there's plenty."

Consider the typical Saturday.

In France, a civilised lunch with friends or family is elegant and restrained. Perhaps a baguette with salad and grilled fish, all sourced fresh from the early morning market after walking there, obviously. One glass of wine, a small dose of existential conversation and an afternoon stroll to soak up the fresh air and sunshine.

In Japan, Saturdays are for errands and family outings. Lunch is light and simple: bento, miso soup, tempura soba or udon, food designed to nourish without slowing the day down.

Meanwhile, in Australia?

Saturday begins with a long, glorious sleep-in, partly because we earned it but mostly because we are recovering from Friday night shenanigans. Eventually we drag ourselves out of bed, reluctantly, and roll straight into Saturday lunch at a Bunnings sausage sizzle. Onions underneath the sausage (safety first), drenched in your sauce of choice and a soft drink to wash it down, all justified because we are going to mow the lawn later, which absolutely counts as exercise.

After that, we reward ourselves for a job well done. More alcohol for the adults, more soft drinks for the kids and most likely a takeaway dinner for all. Perhaps fish and chips because "they'll soak up the alcohol," a comforting lie we've all told ourselves.

Of course, these are broad brushstrokes. Cultures aren't perfect, and no country eats flawlessly. But these patterns exist, and they influence how we eat, move, socialise and think about food.

And the numbers reflect a global shift. As Western fast food has spread, overweight and obesity rates have risen almost everywhere.

Fast food isn't the sole problem. Processed food in general, including cakes, commercial bread, flavoured milk drinks and yoghurts, orange juice, "healthy" muesli bars and most breakfast cereals, tends to be filled with ingredients that are far removed from their natural state. Minimal processing, like chopping, blending or grinding whole foods, is not the issue. The problems arise when foods are altered with additives, sugars, oils and fillers. Avoiding fast food alone is not enough. Checking ingredients and being more discerning when shopping has become essential.

Stricter and more transparent labelling laws would also help. Imagine if packaging showed the percentage of ingredients that were unprocessed. Most people would soon find themselves shopping around the perimeter of the supermarket, because that is where the foods closest to nature are found.

In Australia, the last official reports from 2022 found around 34 percent of adults were overweight and 32 percent were obese (the overweight number only dropped because many people were reclassified into the obese category). Projections suggest these numbers are still climbing.

With Australia now ranking in the top 10 OECD nations for obesity, it's hard to deny how powerfully our environment shapes our habits.

Any long-term way of eating must fit the culture you're living in; otherwise, it becomes just another diet, short-lived, uncomfortable and destined to fall apart the moment real life kicks in. If we want to lose weight and keep it off, our approach must make sense within the Aussie way of living, not work against it.

A big part of modern Australian life is shaped by the cultures we are closest to. We share far more culturally with the US and the UK than we ever have with France or Japan.

From America, we embraced fast food, drive-through restaurants, super-size meal deals and giant gas-guzzling SUVs complete with cup holders big enough for a litre of iced coffee.

From the Brits, we enthusiastically adopted wine o'clock, that magical window between late afternoon and dinner when a glass seems to call your name. Naturally, we improved on the concept, as evidenced on Melbourne Cup Day, the race that stops the nation. Champagne flows with joyous abandon not only trackside, but also at Champagne breakfasts and ladies' lunches across the country, often well before the first race begins at 10:30am... on a Tuesday.

And America, always supportive, handed us the ultimate permission slip:

"It's five o'clock somewhere."

It practically became a national slogan.

Two cultures that don't exactly have stellar track records with weight and health blended seamlessly into our relaxed, sun-soaked Australian lifestyle. It's no surprise we ended up with generous portions, gatherings that revolve around food and alcohol, and easy access to inexpensive, high-calorie foods, much of it woven into our daily routine.

We are products of our environment, one that quietly encourages overeating without us noticing... or more accurately, without us wanting to notice.

And through all of this, the French elegance we never quite adopted, the Japanese discipline we never mastered, the American fast food we absorbed, and the British drinking culture we embraced, Australian women developed a very particular attitude toward weight.

We are not a culture that fears getting fat, panics over a stray kilo, or lives in constant food anxiety. We simply don't view weight as a moral failure, nor should we.

If anything, our approach is almost casual:

"Yeah, I've put on a bit of weight... but it'll come off."

For years, that laid-back confidence serves us well, right up until it doesn't.

ONE

Powders And Diets: The Journey

I was the original guinea pig long before this reset ever existed. Back when I launched Yeppoonie Smoothie in the little coastal town of Yeppoon in Queensland, I tested every blend on myself.

The business started with a simple product idea: healthy, nutritious smoothie powders which are filling, high in fibre and protein and easy to use. I wanted to provide a clean option for people who were busy, tired or simply trying to eat well without overthinking it, people just like me. I was trying to create something nourishing, energising and easy. So I tweaked ingredients, experimented with formulas and paid attention to what genuinely worked. Little by little, the blends took shape.

Documenting this reset felt strangely familiar. I was the guinea pig again, but this time the stakes were different. I needed to know this wasn't just another fad diet. I wanted proof that real change was possible without turning anyone's life inside out. If an approach is overly complicated, rigid, or restrictive, it never lasts, not for a week and certainly not for a month. It must be convenient and blend effortlessly into everyday life. If your new diet plan cannot do that, the method needs adjusting, not you.

My hope is that this gives you tools which you will use long after The Reset is over. You may find some of it familiar: a mash-up of the diets you have tried, mixed with practices that help you look beneath the surface, understand what brought you here, and move forward in a lighter, calmer way.

As a mum and someone inching towards fifty, I see life through a very different lens than I did in my twenties and thirties. Would I tell that younger version of myself to do anything differently? I don't think so. Every choice, from the wise to the questionable, brought me to the here and now. And I've learned that new beginnings don't arrive once a year; they happen daily. If you're here for one, you're in the right place.

And for the record, I am not a doctor, nutritionist, or dietitian. But I am a woman at the helm of a wellness business, and someone who has spent years paying attention to what works in real life as well as in theory. My smoothie powder blends are savoured daily by thousands of Australian women and men, giving me a window into what people struggle with, what they crave, and what genuinely helps.

I am not writing from a laboratory or a clinical setting. I am writing from the place most women actually live: juggling, adjusting, simplifying, experimenting, and discovering what helps them thrive by doing. That, I think, is exactly what sets this reset apart.

It has been seven or eight years since my last deliberate attempt at weight loss. I also use the word *diet* in this book. And yes, I know it is unfashionable in the wellness world, but let us be honest: we all know what it means. We all have an everyday diet; going on one simply means changing what you normally eat. We do not need to tiptoe around the word.

Back then, my entire approach revolved around exercise, and frustratingly it slowed me down. I ate more to fuel the workouts, which left me tired, puffy, and constantly hungry. It always felt like a grind.

These days, I find that if I get my diet in order first, if everything inside is running more smoothly, I naturally want to move. That sluggish, lazy feeling lifts, and a quiet little spark kicks in. Suddenly I am motivated to sort my wardrobe, dust the house, tidy things up... all the little corners of life I have been ignoring.

Once you start cleansing your body, you often feel compelled to cleanse everything else too. And it works in reverse. Anyone who has done a Marie-Kondo-style clean-out knows the sudden urge to clean up your eating afterward.

So when that spark appears, it is an invitation to begin movement and exercise, and walking is the perfect place to start. It is good for both the body and the mind, and gentle enough to do every day.

Of course, I already knew the weight-loss theories. I hear the same questions from Yeppoonie customers every day, including how much they can lose per week and how quickly they can lose it. Regardless of the question, one thing I have learned from developing Yeppoonie blends and losing weight myself is this: biology never lies. Real change happens only when you work with your body, not against it.

I too was ready, yet again, to shed the extra kilos I had accumulated, and it gave me the perfect opportunity to run this experiment properly. Weight creeps up slowly; we turn a blind eye, tell ourselves we will deal with it later, and use alcohol, sugary drinks, and comfort food as emotional fillers, which only compounds the problem.

I didn't gain weight on purpose just so I could write this book, a perfectly reasonable justification for a year of indulgence. The truth is far less glamorous. Those extra kilos were the remnants of business demands, teenage-daughter drama (the payback I always suspected was coming), moving house, moving business premises, setting up a café, then a bar, all while navigating peri- and post-menopause, ageing, and the hormonal fluctuations that come with it. I had become a guinea pig in her prime.

It wasn't until I finally decided to slow down, and the dust settled, that it became clear I needed a reset.

That was the moment I decided to document everything. Yeppoonie customers often asked whether we recommended a weight loss plan. We provided strategies and resets, but nothing all encompassing. I realised the only plan worth sharing is the one I have genuinely lived. If you want to get rich, you ask a rich person. If you want to slim down, you ask someone who has done so and continues to live that way.

The only thing revolutionary about my plan is its simplicity. It requires a kilo of commitment and an ounce of willpower, but after day one... then day two... then day six... it starts to click. Of course, then comes the weekend obstacle course: parties, family meals, and all the usual distractions. But if you treat it as a challenge rather than a punishment, the pressure lifts and it becomes something you can stick to.

And once it became something I could stick to, the rest followed. Fortunately, once I commit, losing weight has never been an issue. The harder part is adjusting my mindset. A clear goal and a deadline make all the difference. With my fiftieth birthday approaching, Christmas Day no less, I set a goal to lose about ten kilos. I say "about" because I truly didn't know the number. I didn't own scales then but ended up buying a set after starting The Reset for "research" purposes. I know my body, I know how I want to look, and I know when I feel comfortable, so that feeling is usually my guide, not the number on the scale.

Aussie women are not scared of a challenge; truthfully, we are not scared of much at all. People overseas imagine Australia as a land crawling with danger, but most of us barely notice the spiders, snakes, sharks, or stingrays. We grow up with them, learn the risks, and then get on with life.

A bit of fat? Not scary.
Lifestyle change? That spooks us.

We do not want to give up the Bunnings sausage sizzle, the big café breakfasts, the beer slabs, or wine cartons. Cutting them out completely feels extreme.

We are practical, straight-talking, and don't tend to fuss. But even with all that no-nonsense strength, the truth is this: any woman can feel thrown by her weight when it comes with constant bloating, puffiness, tiredness, and that heavy, achy, inflamed feeling.

Enter the diet.

This book is not a long-term diet. It is a reset: a way to calm the stomach, steady your energy, quiet the background noise around food, and ease the stubborn belly weight that no amount of kale or cardio ever seems to touch. It is not glamorous, complicated, or trending, but it works because it respects how women actually live. It offers early dinners, simple meals, gentler routines, better sleep, fewer decisions, and less overwhelm. It will also help you learn how to eat in the real world, after any diet or weight-loss solution.

It helps peel back the layers of your life that led you to first accumulate weight and then hold onto it, along with everything that comes with that: inflammation, fatigue, and that familiar sense of heaviness. That, I think, is where this book differs from most.

Before we go any further, I want to address the obvious question that comes up whenever someone writes a weight loss book.
The inevitable response when I said I was writing one was, of course, "Oh, another one. Aren't there enough?"

Enough? Hmm. The diet and weight loss category on Amazon Australia alone shows over 70,000 listings, so yes, there are more than enough. But clearly they are not working if the majority of Australians are now overweight, and that tipping point happened some time ago. Maybe mine will be the one that does. It has certainly made a difference to me, and I am the kind of person who knows within two pages whether a diet book is right for me. From what I have seen, most either take too much away or add too much in, and either way they make life harder. I want to give back and simplify.

If we stopped creating things simply because the world already had a lot of them, nothing meaningful would ever be made.

There is a book I adore called *The Artist's Way* by Julia Cameron. The *New York Times* once called her "the Queen of Change." She takes readers, many of them blocked writers and artists, on a path of self-discovery using journaling and gentle creative practices. Her techniques can reignite a creative light a reader may have thought long extinguished. Elizabeth Gilbert famously said that without *The Artist's Way*, there would be no *Eat Pray Love*.

I like to think this book places you on a similar, parallel path. I do not believe weight problems are solved by simply eating better and doing more cardio. Just as *The Artist's Way* clears creative blockages if you stick with it, I hope this book helps clear the barriers that lead to weight gain and to holding onto weight. Julia Cameron sends you deep within yourself and then back out into the world. I want you to begin by spending real time with yourself in your own space and by addressing the priorities that have been buried while you have taken care of everyone else.

So is it another diet book? I like to think it is more than that, but you will have to read on and decide for yourself.

TWO

You Decide You've Had Enough

Just like weight gain doesn't happen overnight, the decision to tackle weight loss rarely arrives in one lightning-bolt moment. It's usually a long, private argument that starts with:

I need to...
Tomorrow...
After this weekend...
Never again...
Why, oh why?...

Until one day, for no obvious reason, you wake up and decide that today is the day.

I am sure you have had that morning.

You wake up, roll over, place your hand on your stomach and think, "Right. That's it. I've had enough."

You wander into the bathroom, stand in front of the mirror, and examine yourself from every angle, as if you need visual confirmation of what you already know. You do the full scan: poke, prod, lift, turn sideways, assess. A forensic-level investigation.

As if your whole belly pushing out in front when you bend down, and your lower back firing off warning shots as you realise it now takes more effort than it used to, isn't sign enough.

But this time feels different.
This time you are motivated.

And in my case, the clock was ticking (not that clock): the turning-fifty-later-in-the-year clock, which lit a fire under me. I have always found it easier to commit when there is a deadline. We all have one: an upcoming party, a trip overseas, a looming hospital visit, or, horror of horrors, a thirty-year school reunion. Use these deadlines; they are your invisible weight-loss buddies.

So you stand there and make a quiet declaration to yourself: "No more procrastinating. I'm changing things up, and I start today."
Not next Monday.
Not after the next birthday, holiday, breakup, school term or failed date.
Not after the next grocery shop where you swear you will buy chia seeds and still walk out without them.

Right now.
You are simply over it.
You are ready to make a change, and this time, you are sticking to it.

Why Women Hit This Point

It is often a slow build-up of tiny irritations:

Elastic has become your new best friend.
Loose, billowy blouses start creeping in and suddenly you're dressing like your mother (who is eighty-five).
You catch a glimpse in a shop window and think, who is she and why is she shaped like that?
You're sending every online order back because you've gone up two sizes.
You feel like your metabolism packed its bags and left without saying goodbye.

And it is not just about size; it is about comfort.

We want to feel comfortable in our clothes, in our routine, in our own skin. We want our body to feel like it's on our side again, not waging a hormonal cold war.

And yes, deep down we always hope there is an easy solution, but experience tells us otherwise.

So we brace ourselves and start another dreaded diet.

Diets have a special gift: they make you feel like you need to become an upgraded version of yourself just to shift a few stubborn kilos. Suddenly you're meant to juice celery (full disclosure: I do love a homemade green juice), buy supplements from strangers on TikTok, or cook meals requiring twenty-seven ingredients, a mortar and pestle, and superhuman patience.

Meanwhile, life is already full: kids, work, ageing parents, hormones coming and going, bills just coming, birthdays, errands, and the eternal laundry pile. No one wants to reinvent their entire kitchen just to feel better in their jeans.

What We Actually Want

What we really want is live-in staff... but since that is not happening, we want something realistic: a low-stress, everyday way of eating that works on any kind of day. The tired days, the rushed days, the good days, and the days when we would happily outsource dinner.

We want a way of eating that does not demand a bigger budget or a pantry overhaul. One that settles the stomach, evens out the appetite, and steadily trims the weight that has been clinging on like a stalactite for years. Most importantly, we want an approach that fits naturally into the way Australian women already live.

That is what this reset offers: a "she'll-be-right" approach to fat loss that fits around real life, not the other way around.

Your body is not against you; it is simply waiting for the right conditions to let go, and those conditions are far simpler than you have ever been told.

This reset does not begin with a dramatic promise.

It begins with recognising that you are not interested in making dieting a lifelong hobby. You just want your stomach to stop sticking out like you are storing snacks for later, your digestion to settle, your clothes to feel comfortable, your energy to lift, and your body to finally feel like it is working with you again.

THREE

The Reasons

Before we move into the mechanics of The Reset, let's quickly look at the most common reasons behind that now-resident weight gain:

- hormones influence appetite
- stress influences digestion
- sleep influences cravings
- inflammation influences bloating

Most Aussie women tick all four boxes because everyday life is busy, full, emotional, messy, and wildly unpredictable.

And women over 30 (not just 40) begin shifting internally in ways that make the middle a little more stubborn. You don't need a science lesson; just one simple idea:

Your body hangs onto extra weight when it feels unsafe, overloaded, inflamed, or out of balance. Like a hoarder, it will hold anything it considers useful: fat, fluid, energy.

Your Body Isn't Against You: It's Sending a Message

Don't think of your bulges as the enemy; think of them as information.

Your body is saying:

- "I'm tired."
- "I'm stressed."

• "I can't keep up."
• "Stop confusing me."
• "Please, for the love of God, stop feeding me ten different things at once."

Your body isn't broken; it is coping.
And the moment you stop ignoring those messages, your body begins to shift. It will not happen overnight, but it will happen.

This reset is about:
• simple meals
• predictable structure
• fewer decisions
• greater ease

The body thrives on calm.

Here is what people generally gloss over:

The female body is incredibly sensitive to stress, not just the emotional kind but any load that feels too much. You can be eating well and still hold belly fat because elevated cortisol tells your body to store energy. You might not feel stressed in any obvious way, but your body can be quietly running on alert.

Late nights, conflict, over committing, rushing, too much coffee, too much exercise, busy schedules, even tiny daily irritations, your system logs all of it like files in a cabinet. When the cabinet is full, the belly becomes the storage unit.

The more women push through pretending they are fine, the more the stomach swells as a warning signal. Your body is not punishing you; it is trying to slow you down.

Inflammation: It Sneaks Up on You

Women underestimate how quickly inflammation builds and the impact it has. You can eat decent food and still carry fluid, puffiness, and that heavy-stomach feeling simply because your system is irritated. Common triggers include:

- irregular eating
- lack of sleep
- hormonal changes
- dehydration
- certain oils
- alcohol
- processed foods
- too many different foods in one day

Often the belly shows it first, visually, long before anything feels wrong. Sometimes it shows up as niggling aches, stiff joints, or fullness through the face. This isn't your age catching up with you, even though it's easy to assume that.

Digestion Slows Long Before Women Notice

Many women have sluggish digestion and assume it is normal to feel heavy after meals or to bloat by mid-afternoon. It is not normal; it is just common. When I follow this plan, none of that happens.

When digestion slows, the body becomes cautious. It will not release fat because it does not feel stable. Sometimes that belly bulge is simply your gut saying, "I need a break," not "you need to punish yourself with another strict diet."

When digestion calms, the belly responds quickly.

Hormones Join the Party (Invited or Not)

Hormonal fluctuations start earlier than most women expect. Progesterone begins to decline in the mid-thirties, stress hormones become more reactive and the body becomes slightly less insulin sensitive, all long before periods become irregular.

When the body becomes less insulin sensitive, blood sugar spikes become more common. Insulin's job is to move glucose from your bloodstream into your cells, but when your cells do not respond as well, your body must release more insulin to get the same job done. If it cannot keep up, your blood sugar stays higher for longer after meals. This leads to bigger spikes, more energy crashes and more fat stored around the belly. Midlife hormones and higher cortisol levels make this even more noticeable because they further reduce insulin sensitivity and raise blood sugar on their own. This is why a low-GI way of eating is useful for every woman.

These shifts influence:

- appetite
- fluid retention
- cravings
- sleep
- mood
- how your body stores fat

Your body updates its operating system as you age, and the stomach is the first app to glitch.

You can eat the same foods you have always eaten and get totally different results simply because your hormonal landscape has shifted. And when your hormones are already shifting, this same-old approach only adds to the confusion.

Too Many Plans, Too Much Input

Women collect diet advice like we collect reusable shopping bags: random, mismatched, overflowing.

A bit of keto.

A bit of fasting.

A podcast snack rule.

A TikTok gut cleanse.

A paleo email newsletter.

Individually, none are bad, but mashed together they confuse the body. Strip back the clutter and your stomach relaxes.

When Life Gets Full

There comes a point where you realise you haven't had a moment to yourself in daylight in... who knows how long. Between school runs, work deadlines, family dramas, and general adulting, your body quietly slips down the priority list.

Women extinguish spot fires all day. We manage emotions that aren't ours and often carry the additional mental load of multiple people: family, friends, colleagues. While we're doing all of that, the body absorbs everything like a sponge. It never begins with an obvious meltdown; it starts with a whisper, the kind that's easy to miss in the middle of everyday chaos.

Most of us don't hear it at all. And even when we do notice the signs, we often ignore them and keep going. But the body doesn't forget. It waits, it compensates, and eventually, when it can't keep up any longer, it pushes back. Suddenly:

- you are exhausted
- your digestion feels unpredictable
- your cravings ramp up

- your sleep goes haywire
- your belly looks different
- your patience evaporates
- and life feels heavier than it did a month ago

This is accumulation. Years of pushing, juggling, overthinking and functioning with a sleep deficit. Women keep going regardless, but the body keeps the score, and eventually everything catches up with you.

Women Survive on Adrenaline Longer Than Anyone Realises

Women can soldier on with four hours of sleep and sheer determination. You can run a household and appear serene, even while you're paddling frantically beneath the surface. Women are masters of looking fine. But adrenaline was never designed to keep us running forever.

When it's high, the body switches into survival mode: digestion slows, fat loss stops, hormones wobble. And the "danger" can be something as simple as a chaotic week or an inbox full of passive-aggressive emails.

When the body doesn't feel safe, it hangs on for dear life. That's why women can be doing everything right and still see nothing shift.

The Emotional Load

Women also absorb emotional weight that is not theirs:

- overwhelmed kids
- partners carrying their own worries
- family tensions
- friends in crisis
- the mental load of preventing problems before they happen

Emotional labour has a physical cost.

Your body responds to emotional strain the same way it responds to anything demanding: it shifts into protection mode and starts hoarding.

And Then There's Wine, Comfort Food and Late-Night Grazing

Women do not emotionally eat because they lack discipline; they do it because they are spent. Wine becomes the signal that the day is finally over; carbs take the edge off the mental load; and snacks feel like a small reward for simply getting through.

It might look like indulgence from the outside, but most of the time it is simply a woman coping with the day she has just had. The real issue is not the food at all; it is the rhythm your body has been trying to follow and the fact that it keeps getting disrupted. It is the inconsistency, the stop-start pattern that never lets your system settle, and the split-second choices you make when you are running on empty and reacting rather than choosing.

These tiny, almost invisible patterns influence how the body functions long before most women realise what is happening. And then, almost without warning, you reach a point where you feel completely at capacity.

This is where The Reset becomes necessary. It is time to recalibrate and give your body some predictability again. This helps it feel safe enough to release what it has been holding onto: fat, fluid, inflammation, tension, stress chemicals, and brain fog. This moment is the turning point.

Keep this in mind: your belly isn't stubborn because you are. It is responding to a body that has been stretched in ten different directions and is simply doing its best to cope. Once you create a steady rhythm, your stomach responds quickly, often faster than most women expect. A calm body lets go. A reactive body holds on.

I will never forget something I learned long before I ever cared about hormones, digestion, or stress.

When I was pregnant with my first daughter, I attended neonatal classes at the Royal Women's Hospital in Melbourne. Our group was blessed with an inspiring instructor. She was a midwife and a mother of four, and she told us she had personally been through every kind of birth imaginable. Then she offered a line that has stayed with me ever since:

"Open mind, open body."

She meant it literally for labour, but it applies everywhere.

When the mind unclenches, the body follows.
When you feel safe, calm, supported, the body releases.
When you tense, brace, or push through, the body protects.

It is the same with weight, digestion, cravings, and belly fat.

Your body is not being stubborn; it is simply responding to the signal you are sending. And the good news?

You are about to learn a rhythm that finally gives your body what it has been asking for.

Not French, not Japanese, not Mediterranean, but an approach that is uniquely Australian and designed for our everyday reality.

FOUR

The Mechanics

People love to say weight-loss attempts fail because women lack discipline or motivation. They are wrong. Women have more discipline than half the planet combined. We run homes, raise kids, hold down jobs or run companies, manage crises, handle illnesses, and keep everyone else alive and functioning, usually without acknowledgement or a day off. Our minds track every appointment (well, almost), every bill, every birthday, and every tiny detail no one else even notices.

When things start to go off the rails, it is almost never a discipline problem. For most women, it is overload that takes us out. When your nervous system is frayed, your mind is cluttered, your hormones feel unsettled and your life is being held together by caffeine and responsibility, willpower is not going to save you. It is not because you are weak; it is because you are running on empty. You do not need more motivation. You need simplicity: a plan that is not demanding, high-maintenance, or designed for someone with a live-in chef and zero responsibilities.

This reset works because it takes the mental weight out of food. When the constant chatter stops, progress finally starts. Many women feel a wave of relief the moment they commit to beginning a new diet plan, and that feeling is often the first sign that the body is ready. Some even feel lighter before changing a single thing they eat, simply because the exhausting internal negotiation has finally ended. No more "I'll start next week." No more bargaining with yourself.

The decision is made and things begin to shift almost at once. You wake up clearer. You prepare food without the usual frenzy. You stop stumbling because you have finally chosen one clear path instead of twenty competing ones. The Reset begins long before your plate changes; it begins the moment your mind quiets and you stop arguing with yourself.

Why It Gets Easier

Once your body receives a predictable rhythm, it responds quickly. Hunger evens out, cravings settle, and energy stops crashing. This is your physiology finally getting what it has been asking for: consistency.

Diets do not fail because women are lazy; they fail because the lifestyle cost is ridiculous. If your plan requires gourmet meals, hours of prep, exotic ingredients, spreadsheets, or a complete shift in who you are, it will not survive a normal week, let alone a demanding one.

Your eating style must work when you are tired, emotional, travelling, rushing, or simply sick of being in the kitchen. If it cannot survive real life, it is not the right plan.

This is why simplicity is not restrictive; it is the only thing that works long-term. It is also why I love smoothies and why I created Yeppoonie: slipping a pile of nutrition into one easy glass.

The Surprising Power of Doing Less

Women think they need a full transformation to feel better. They do not. They just need to stop doing so bloody much, a lesson I learned the hard way.

When you simplify food, you calm down. When your body knows what is coming, it relaxes. When digestion is not under strain, your stomach naturally settles. When your days have a predictable rhythm, your hormones follow that lead. And when food is no longer taking up so much space in your mind, everything feels lighter. Doing less works because your body is no longer fighting constant disruption.

You are about to learn a method that is refreshingly straightforward, and that is exactly why it works. And here is the best part: you do not need to combine it with exercise if you do not want to or cannot right now, although regular movement, when it is part of your everyday way of life, is encouraged.

Rhythm Matters More Than Food

Most programs skip the most important truth: the rhythm matters more than the food. Read that again.

You can eat the healthiest ingredients in the world, but if your pattern is unpredictable, your body still feels burdened. And you can eat simple, grounding meals, but if your rhythm is consistent, your body responds beautifully.

Rhythm is the secret behind The Reveal Phase, not food alone, not restriction, not punishing workouts on a treadmill. Deep down, people know when they are out of rhythm, but sometimes it is hard to find the beat again. The structure in this reset puts you back in sync.

Patterns Over Variety

Your body thrives with fewer surprises. When it has a sense of what is coming, digestion improves, and once digestion improves, your appetite becomes more stable. A stable appetite naturally lowers cravings, and lower cravings reduce inflammation. With less inflammation, the body finally feels safe enough to release stored fat. This is not about eating the same thing forever; it is about short-term simplicity that creates long-term stability.

Calm Creates Progress

Modern society has long associated progress with intensity and hard work. In wellness, this often translates into more rules, more restriction, and more effort. But when your body is overstimulated, it does not want intensity. It wants relief.

The Reset is essentially the declutter button for your physiology. It removes the fuss, the noise, and the complicated instructions that only make life harder. If a plan demands perfection or constant mental effort, it eventually collapses, not because you failed, but because the plan was unrealistic to begin with. You do not need to love cooking, and you do not need to become a fitness addict. You do not need a brand-new pantry or a brand-new identity. What you need is a structure that feels manageable on your best day and still within reach on your worst; a simple structure you can follow consistently.

Not a Starvation Plan

You will eat a little less than you're accustomed to, but you will not starve. The body adapts far more quickly than most women expect. You will still eat real food that genuinely supports digestion and reduces inflammation. You will feel full. You will have your coffee. Dinner will stay simple and early. Nothing about this reset fights your physiology; it works with it.

If you are used to large portions, daily French fries, ice-cream after dinner, muffins with your coffee or constant snacking, it may feel uncomfortable at first. That does not mean it is wrong for you; it means your body is adjusting. Give it time, reach for the healthy snacks you already have and you will settle into the rhythm.

During my own reset, I experimented with very low-calorie days because I find them helpful in short bursts. But extremely low intake is not sustainable. I learned that quickly. Headaches, nausea, and fatigue are not how I want to live. Those symptoms showed me exactly where the line was. I also used the calorie-burn data from my smartwatch as a general guide for a safe intake.

Everyone is different. What works for one woman may not work for another, which is why I encourage you to use tools like TDEE calculators as guides, not commandments.

One thing I rediscovered, especially after having gestational diabetes years ago, is how much better I feel when my eating is steadier and simpler: lower sugar, low-GI meals, predictable rhythms, and calmer digestion. Calorie counting was not something I even considered, because when you choose the right foods, lower calories become part of the equation automatically. That experience shaped many of the principles behind this reset and even influenced the Yeppoonie blends themselves.

The beauty of this approach is how natural it feels once the rhythm clicks into place. I have never understood why so many diet books complicate everything with endless recipes and rigid structures. The trick is keeping things simple. Variety might be the spice of life, but not during a reset.

Simplicity carries you through the days you are low on energy, the days that feel heavy, and the nights when preparing dinner feels like too much effort. When you are not juggling complicated recipes or cooking multiple versions of the same meal, everything becomes lighter. You can still cook what your family loves; you just keep your own plate uncomplicated.

This is not a dramatic transformation.

It is a gentle structure, one that soothes digestion, steadies appetite, quiets the mental clutter around food, and lets your body finally relax. And once that happens, many things begin to blossom.

Why Repetition Works

Repetition reduces the mental load. It gives your digestion a break, stabilises your hormones, and prepares your body for the Reveal Phase. Once things settle, the bloating drops, cravings fade, and appetite regulates, you will have more flexibility. But first, we simplify. This repetition is not forever; it is a reset.

In the next chapter we move into the actual plan: what you eat, when you eat, and how the rhythm works.

FIVE
The Reset

This chapter outlines The Reset: the foods, the timing, and the structure that will shape your days. You could skip straight here and begin at once, but it genuinely helps to understand the triggers behind weight gain and why this rhythm works so well. A little context makes the whole process feel more logical, and therefore easier to stick to.

If anyone asks what you're doing, the simplest explanation is this:

"It's a reset built around lower calories/kilojoules (but not extreme), low-GI eating, gentle intermittent fasting, and light movement."

I recommend following it for thirty days to give your body time to settle, but once you're in the rhythm and start seeing results, you'll naturally keep going until you reach the weight that feels good. Most women know instinctively when they've reached that point.

And even afterwards, you can return to The Reset whenever you need it, for a few days, a week, or a quick tune-up when habits slip. I keep this structure as my everyday routine now. It's no longer "a reset"; it simply became my baseline.

The Simple Daily Structure Outline

Throughout The Reset, a Day Has Three Phases, Not Three Meals.

Most diets talk about meals: breakfast, lunch, dinner, as if they're purely about food. But in this reset, we're not organising your day around eating;

we're organising it around physiology. That's why I use the word phases. Each phase has a purpose beyond simply "having a meal." One phase steadies your hormones for the day ahead, one keeps your blood sugar stable and your digestion light, and one sets your system up for overnight fat burning. When you think in phases instead of meals, you stop focusing on "what to eat next" and start focusing on how each part of the day supports your metabolism, nervous system, and appetite regulation.

This structure works because it aligns with your natural hormone patterns, appetite cycles, digestion, and the way the female body prefers to run once it's not being pushed and overstimulated.

It mirrors the philosophy behind the Yeppoonie Smoothie blends: Good Morning, Good Afternoon and Good Evening. Each one supports a different part of the day rather than being just another meal replacement in a glass.

In this book I talk about women, and The Reset is especially beneficial for women in their mid-thirties and beyond. But younger women, and men too, will benefit from it.

Here's how the phases work:

Phase One: The Morning Calm

The goal in this phase is to keep appetite steady and blood sugar flat. Your first meal should feel grounding rather than stimulating. It must have enough protein, enough fibre, and nothing sugary or spiky. This sets the tone for the whole day and prevents that mid-morning "searching for something" feeling.

Snacks?

If you need a snack, the morning is the best place for it, as this is when your body metabolises food the most efficiently.

Phase Two: The Midday Nourish

This is where you feed your body clean, supportive fuel. You're stable from the morning, your digestion is ready, and your energy systems can use nutrients efficiently. A simple, balanced lunch keeps your afternoon stable, prevents the common 3pm to 4pm slump, and as you are adequately nourished, it also reduces evening cravings. Think of it as topping up the tank just enough, without pushing it into overflow.

Snacks?

If you feel hungry in the afternoon, a light, protein-rich mini-snack can help: yoghurt, eggs, kimchi, radishes, or a small handful of nuts. Keep it simple and calming. By late afternoon, insulin sensitivity drops, cravings rise, and the body becomes more likely to store food than burn it, which is why late-day snacking works against you.

Phase Three: The Evening Restore

This phase is all about giving your body the conditions it needs to release, repair, and settle overnight. Eating early and lightly allows your digestive system to wind down, your inflammation to ease, and your overnight metabolic patterns to work in your favour. You're essentially creating a gentle internal environment where your nervous system regulates, your hormones rebalance, and your overnight fat-burning signals can switch on without interruption.

Snacks?

A warming caffeine-free drink is best.

Your Nourishing Food Structure For Each Phase

First, a note on portions and calories:

Exact serving sizes and calorie or kilojoule counts are not specified in all the following meals by design. This nutritional reset emphasises satiety rather than restriction or excessive monitoring. Individual needs will vary and may even change throughout the day. By tuning into your body's hunger signals, which will be discussed later, you will naturally determine the quantities that support your weight management goals.

As a starting point, aim for small, palm-sized portions from each food group at every meal (for example, chicken as one group and vegetables as another), and adjust these amounts as needed.

Serving suggestions are designed for one person and you can multiply the ingredients easily if you are cooking for more.

It helps to eat or drink slowly, pause halfway, and aim to stop when you feel comfortably satisfied rather than overfull. Every woman's appetite is different, especially as hormones shift. Trusting your body to guide you creates a far more stable, predictable rhythm, than counting numbers on a page ever could. This approach keeps things simple, sustainable, and grounded in real life.

If you are interested in tracking calories/kilojoules there is a table in Appendix C at the end of this book.

Phase 1: The Morning Calm

(*Keep your metabolism in a good mood*)

Breakfast Timing and Purpose

I prefer to eat breakfast between **8am and 10am**.

This naturally gives me a gentle 14–16 hour overnight fast, depending on when I eat dinner. I find this window easy to tolerate.

If you need to eat breakfast earlier for any reason, adjust all your meal times accordingly. Try to maintain these times each day where you can. The Reset is meant to work around your lifestyle, not the other way around.

Keep breakfast simple and protein-plus-fibre forward, and it will help stabilise blood sugar, reduce morning grazing, and keep your appetite calm.

The reward of a decent breakfast is less cravings throughout the day.

Two Suggested Morning Options:

OPTION 1:

Wake-up Smoothie (Protein + Fibre)

A simple morning smoothie works beautifully.

Blend in blender:

- 250-300ml unsweetened almond milk (or preferred milk/water)
- 1 scoop high-protein powder or Yeppoonie Smoothie powder of choice
- 1–2 tsp of psyllium or ground flax if not using Yeppoonie
- 1–2 tsp unsweetened Greek yoghurt
- 3–4 berries and ¼ banana only (if needed for taste and density)
- Add a shot of coffee if you desire

Keeps morning sugar extremely low and fibre to keep you full

OPTION 2:

Two Eggs Plus Boosters

Eggs give your brain and hormones the stability they need in the morning.

Boiled, poached, or scrambled. You can add some rocket, herbs, kimchi to have on the side.

Fibre and protein boosters:

- 1–2 tbsp Greek yoghurt
- ½ avocado
- A handful of spinach (cooked is much higher in fibre)

A healthy way to enjoy a cooked breakfast without the residual heaviness.

OPTION 3:

Overnight Oats (or morning oats if you forgot to soak)

Low GI & Gentle on Digestion.

Half a cup of raw oats soaked overnight in water to lower the GI and make them more digestible.
In the morning, serve with almond milk, a small amount of fruit (such as berries or pawpaw), and a spoon of Greek yoghurt. Sprinkle with half a teaspoon of cinnamon.

Add-ons (optional):

- Hemp Seeds
- One teaspoon of chia seeds
- A few crushed almonds

Overnight oats give you slow, steady energy. A great natural source of soluble fibre.

Breakfast Variations:

You can season things however you like: a sprinkle of herbs, a squeeze of lemon, or a drizzle of olive oil. These breakfasts are flexible, so feel free to mix and match similar ingredients. Keep it simple and make what feels right for you today.

1. **Omelette Fix**

A simple two-egg omelette cooked with minimal oil and filled with spinach, mushrooms, onion and capsicum.

2. **Cottage Cheese Plate**

Half a cup of cottage cheese served with cherry tomatoes, sliced cucumber, basil and a quarter of an avocado, drizzle of olive oil (or similar) plus a teaspoon of LSA for extra fibre and satiety.

3. **Greek Yoghurt Bowl**

3/4 cup of Greek yoghurt mixed with cinnamon to taste, one teaspoon of chia seeds, some berries and chopped pear for crunch. Sprinkle with LSA (available in health section of supermarkets or health food stores).

4. **Protein Scramble**

Two eggs scrambled together with 50–70g of cooked chicken breast, tuna or tofu, garlic and a handful of spinach.

5. **Avocado & Egg Plate**

Two eggs (any style) served with sliced avocado and a handful of fresh salad greens for a green satisfying breakfast.

6. **Cottage Cheese, Apple Cinnamon & LSA Bowl**

Half a cup of cottage cheese mixed with chopped green apple, half a teaspoon of cinnamon and a teaspoon of LSA. A high-protein, high-fibre breakfast that keeps you full, calm and grounded all morning.

7. **Simple Scrambled Tofu Plate**

Soft scrambled tofu cooked with a little turmeric, onion and spinach for a warm, protein-rich plant-based option.

8. **Smoked Salmon & Cucumber Stack**

Smoked salmon layered with thin cucumber slices and a squeeze of lemon for a refreshing, high-protein breakfast. Add a few slices of avocado, a spoon of cottage cheese, a handful of cherry tomatoes, and a boiled egg on the side for extra fullness and balance.

9. **Warm Fruits & Yoghurt Cup**

Greek yoghurt folded through gently stewed apple, warmed berries and a pinch of cinnamon for a cosy yoghurt alternative. Sprinkle with LSA.

10. **Mushroom & Herb Egg White Omelette**

A 3–4 egg white omelette filled with sautéed mushrooms and fresh herbs for a lighter but still protein-forward option. Mix in half a teaspoon of nutritional yeast for added flavour and a gentle nutrition boost.

11. **Protein Bite Plate**

A boiled egg paired with a small portion of cottage cheese, avocado slices, cherry tomatoes and cucumber for a quick, no-fuss breakfast plate.

12. **Simple Banana & Yoghurt Bowl**

Greek yoghurt topped with a few slices of banana and cinnamon for mornings when you want something soft, mild and easy. Sprinkle with LSA.

A Word on Coffee

Coffee Options That Work on The Reset

There are plenty of reset-friendly choices:

- Long black / Americano: best option (zero sugar, low milk)
- Macchiato: just a dash of milk, still low-impact
- Piccolo latte: tiny but satisfying
- Flat white / latte /Cappuccino (small): keep it simple, no syrups
- Cold brew (unsweetened): smooth, strong, no sugar crash

Best to avoid:

- Large oversized milky coffees
- Syrups
- Frappes
- Milky iced drinks
- Sweetened almond milk
- Coffee + pastry combos

The key is small, simple and unsweetened, morning only. Changing from large to small coffee can seem drastic, but once the caffeine kicks in you barely notice the smaller size.

Why no coffee after about 2pm is best

After mid-afternoon, your natural cortisol begins to rise again as part of your circadian rhythm, especially if you're an early riser (around 6–7am). That rise is normal and helps keep you alert for the rest of the day, but adding caffeine on top of it can exaggerate the effect.

Late or excessive caffeine leads to lighter, more disrupted sleep and a tendency to hold onto stubborn belly fat.

I usually have mine after breakfast, and it serves as my mid-meal snack.

Phase 2: The Midday Nourish

(*The anti-bloat, anti-craving, metabolism-soothing phase*)

Lunch Timing and Purpose

Lunch falls anywhere between **12pm and 2pm.**

Again, there's no rigid time, just a predictable mid-day anchor that feeds your body without spiking it. This spacing from breakfast helps stabilise insulin, supports better mood regulation, and prevents the 3pm slump.

Lunch MUST be simple. This is where we often accidentally sabotage ourselves by overthinking. In the middle of the day, we need sustained nourishment rather than "diet food." Think grounding, low-GI, protein-rich meals, which keep energy smooth through the afternoon.

The goal here is easy digestion, stable blood sugar, and zero decision fatigue.

The best option?

A Protein Smoothie of Choice

Blend:

- 250ml-300ml unsweetened almond milk (or preferred milk/water)
- ⅓ cup frozen berries + banana (combined)
- 1 spoon unsweetened Greek yoghurt
- Yeppoonie Smoothie scoop of powder, or your protein powder of choice
- 1 tsp psyllium or ground flax if not using Yeppoonie

Why it works:

- Predictable calories

- High fibre
- Low inflammation
- No insulin spikes
- No digestive stress
- No decisions required
- No afternoon cravings

For many women, bloating reduces within days.

Lunch Variations (if not having a smoothie):

1. Chicken Bowl

A light, satisfying bowl made with 100g of lightly cooked chicken, a generous serve of steamed vegetables, and a simple dressing of olive oil with balsamic vinegar, or soy sauce with chilli flakes and a squeeze of lime for a different flavour profile.

2. Tuna or Tofu Salad Bowl

A refreshing lunch made with a small tin of tuna (or a portion of tofu) tossed with cucumber, tomato, lettuce, leafy greens such as spinach or rocket, sliced onion, a drizzle of olive or your preferred oil and apple cider or balsamic vinegar.

3. Smoked Salmon Plate

One boiled egg paired with about 50g of smoked salmon, a generous bowl of fresh greens and a quarter of an avocado.

4. Veggie Soup with Protein

A warm, broth-based vegetable soup to which you can add chicken, a boiled egg, or tofu for balance and satiety.

5. Greek Yoghurt Plate

Ideal for smaller appetites: half a cup of Greek yoghurt paired with a selection of fresh vegetables such as cucumber, tomato, capsicum strips, celery sticks, radishes, snow peas or baby spinach, finished with a drizzle of olive oil and season to taste.

6. Garden Salad with healthy fats

A simple garden salad with mixed greens, ripe avocado, and a handful of nuts gives you slow, steady-release energy. Combine two cups of greens with cucumber and cherry tomatoes, add half an avocado, and toss through a small handful of almonds or walnuts. Finish with a drizzle of preferred oil and a squeeze of lemon. Add apple cider or balsamic vinegar if you wish.

It's light, nourishing, and keeps your afternoon comfortable and balanced.

Optional: salmon, mackerel, or sardines–add to your Garden Salad for an extra boost of healthy fats.

7. Quick Chicken & Greens Plate

Leftover chicken breast served chilled with spinach, cucumber and a squeeze of lemon for a simple, no-cook morning meal.

8. Leftover veggie bowl

Steam a medley of veggies from the fridge or use last night's leftovers. Add a dollop of cottage cheese and your protein of choice or enjoy it as is. Finish with cracked pepper or fresh herbs if you like.

Phase 3: The Evening Restore

(*When inflammation drops and fat-burning switches on*)

Dinner Timing and Purpose

I aim to eat dinner between **5pm and 7pm**.

I encourage this rhythm because an early evening meal supports steadier digestion, deeper sleep, and better overnight fat-burning. Once dinner is done, the kitchen is closed for the night. If I feel like something warm, I'll have a herbal tea or a cup of warm almond milk with cinnamon and chicory powder (or any caffeine-free evening drink, avoiding cocoa, as it does contain caffeine). I steer clear of dessert, sugar, snacks, and the mindless grazing that creeps in after dinner.

I also let the house wind down: softer lighting, quieter energy, and a gentle evening routine. It's incredibly calming for adults, and it helps guide children into a bedtime rhythm too. This quiet stretch of the evening sets the scene for your body to do its real work, repairing, restoring and releasing while you slumber blissfully unaware.

Dinner Ideas:

Lean Protein + Vegetables

Examples:

1. Chicken & Greens Plate

Tender chicken grilled or shallow fried and served with steamed cabbage, brussels sprouts and broccoli, finished with a light drizzle of olive oil and pepper, plus a dollop of mustard on the side.

2. Fresh Tuna Salad Bowl

A small tin of tuna paired with tomato, onion, cucumber on a bed of crisp lettuce, dressed simply with Apple Cider vinegar and olive or alternative oil.

3. Savoury Omelette & Greens

A warm, protein-rich omelette folded through with mushroom, onion and sautéed greens of choice.

4. Oven-Roasted Chicken & Colourful Veg

Juicy roasted chicken served alongside a medley of cooked colourful vegetables, think capsicum, onion and tomato, finished with a drizzle of olive oil.

5. Hearty Protein Soup Bowl

A soothing bone broth-based soup with egg, tofu, chicken or lean beef, plus a mix of vegetables, ideal for using up anything nearing the end of its life.

6. Tofu & Veggie Stir-Fry

Tofu tossed with cooked vegetables and a spoon of red chilli paste, finished with just enough light coconut cream to coat without drowning it.

7. Lemon Chicken Bowl

Chicken strips tossed with garlic, lemon juice, and pepper, served with steamed zucchini and green beans. Drizzle with olive oil and finish with cracked pepper for a bright, simple, digestion-friendly dinner.

8. Thai-Inspired Fish

A fillet of white fish gently cooked with lemongrass, ginger, and lime, finished with fresh coriander. Serve with lightly stir-fried or steamed broccoli, snow peas, carrot, and chopped cabbage for a light, aromatic meal. Finish with lime and fresh chilli for a bright, zingy flavour.

9. Egg & Greens

Two eggs, scrambled, poached or as a quick omelette, paired with sautéed or steamed greens for an easy, protein-rich option.

10. Beef Bone Broth & Vegetable Soup

A comforting bowl made with beef bone broth (I love Nutra Organics broth powder), sliced beef, onion, garlic, and mushrooms, plus any vegetables you need to use up, leek, cabbage, celery, a small carrot, or even a small low-GI potato.

11. Simple Stir-Fry

A quick stir-fry made with minimal oil, plenty of mixed vegetables, and your protein of choice. Keep the condiments light and low in sugar so the flavours stay clean and supportive of your reset. Finish with fresh herbs, lime, or cracked pepper if you like.

12. Grilled Chicken on Fresh Garden Salad

Refreshing and light, grilled or pan-fried chicken, chopped into bite-sized pieces, served on a mixed garden salad with onion, cherry tomato halves and red onion. Drizzle with Apple Cider Vinegar and oil of choice and cracked black pepper.

13. Curry of Choice

Use your preferred curry spice mix: Thai, Indian, or Japanese. Keep it simple by skipping the rice and cream. Load it with vegetables and your choice of protein for a warm, satisfying, low-GI meal.

The Snack Strategy

Snacking can slow progress for most women over 40. However, this isn't a starvation plan. If you're genuinely hungry, not bored or emotional, have something small and sensible:

Always remember, **a snack is a bridge, not a new meal.**

Most women find their hunger stabilises after a few days and snacks naturally disappear, but some days you'll need one or two. That's fine.

Blood-sugar–friendly snacks:

✓ 8–10 raw almonds

Small serve only, to keep insulin stable.

✓ Kimchi–great as a snack or with a meal

Spicy, zingy, and great for your gut.

✓ Radishes or cucumber slices with a teaspoon of hummus

Crunchy, refreshing, zero spike.

✓ Cucumber slices with lemon and cracked black pepper

✓ Radishes with a drizzle of olive oil and a pinch of sea salt

✓ Green cold-pressed juice made from:

- spinach
- cucumber
- celery
- ginger
- ¼ carrot for sweetness only

No apple, orange, pineapple or beetroot.

✓ 1 boiled egg

A perfect biological hunger fix. Keep a few pre-boiled in their shells in the fridge for easy grab-and-go.

✓ 1 green apple

Another great hunger fix, and you'll genuinely relish your apple a day. Just keep it to one piece of fruit daily, so if you've already had fruit with your breakfast or smoothie, choose another snack instead.

✓ 1 pear

Also a great hunger fix and your gut will love you as it's a great fibre source. As per the apple regarding one fruit serve per day.

✓ Herbal tea

Warmth kills most cravings.

✓ Mixed seeds

Pumpkin Seeds are a nutritious snack and handy to have on hand. You can fry to toast them too, no oil or salt needed.

Note:
If you're needing snacks all day, it possibly means:

- you need more fibre and protein at breakfast and lunch
- you had too much caffeine
- dinner was too late
- you're overtired or over-stressed

Your body is signalling, listen to it.

The Good Fats

Not all fat is unwanted, and no woman should be afraid of healthy fat.

In fact, these are some of the most supportive foods you can include in your daily routine. They steady your appetite, steady your hormones, support your brain, balance your blood sugar, and deliver essential omega-3 and omega-6 fatty acids, the kind your body can't make on its own. These omegas help regulate inflammation, support hormone production, nourish your skin, sharpen your thinking, and keep you fuller for longer.

A small amount is all you need and they can make any meal more satisfying without derailing your reset. Healthy fats keep cravings low, energy stable, and digestion smoother.

Here are some simple ways to add healthy fats to your meals (remember, you only need a little, think of them as boosters):

Avocado Slices

A quarter to half an avocado added to eggs, salads or bowls provides gentle, stable energy without spiking blood sugar.

Avocado Herb Dip

Mash one ripe avocado with a tablespoon or two of olive oil, a handful of chopped herbs and a squeeze of lemon or lime. Season to taste and adjust the olive oil until you reach your preferred texture.

Extra Virgin Olive, Avocado or Hemp Seed Oil Drizzle

Drizzle lightly over cooked vegetables or salads to add healthy fats which support hormones and help you stay fuller for longer.

Tahini spoon

Stirring a small amount through vegetables or drizzled over eggs gives a creamy, savoury richness without sugar.

Almond butter swipe

A thin spread on cucumber or celery sticks offers a satisfying, quick hit of healthy fats.

Hemp seed sprinkle

A tablespoon over salads or omelettes adds healthy fats and minerals, with almost no flavour impact.

Chia or ground flax mix-in

Add to yoghurt, smoothies or oats to add fibre + healthy fats that help with satiety and digestion.

Small handful (4-5) of Walnuts

A classic, quick stabiliser when you're genuinely hungry in between meals.

The Daily Structure (A Sample Day)

Breakfast (7am–10am ideal)

- 2 boiled eggs with fresh spinach, 1 cherry tomato, sliced cucumber
- 2–3 tsp Greek yoghurt with sprinkle of cinnamon
- Small coffee

Lunch (12pm–2pm ideal)

- A low-sugar, fibre + protein–rich smoothie
  (or chicken and salad if preferred)

Dinner (5pm–7pm ideal)

- Lean beef sliced into thin strips and lightly pan-fried
- Steamed vegetables
- A spoon of mustard
- Herbal tea afterwards

Snacks

- None, or optional low-impact choices if needed

Drinks

- Water
- Herbal tea
- Coffee (morning only)

Movement

- Light walk or stretching at any time of day
  (avoid too close to bedtime)

Bedtime

- Ideally between 9:30pm and 10:30pm

Foods To ENJOY or AVOID During The 30-Day Reset

Foods to Avoid During the 30-Day Reset:

These foods tend to trigger insulin spikes, inflammation, cravings, and bloating:

- **Bread** (If you must, choose dense low-GI rye or *true* sourdough. No more than **2 thin slices** in a day and not every day.)
- **Pasta** (If needed, choose wholegrain/low-GI and keep the serve small.)
- **Rice** (Limit to brown rice and keep servings modest.)
- **Potatoes** (Choose low-GI varieties and limit to **one small/baby potato** with a meal.)
- **Sweets & pastries**
- **Biscuits**
- **Chocolate**
- **Juice** (Only homemade, cold-pressed green vegetable juice is okay—e.g. cucumber, celery, leafy greens, lemon, ginger.)
- **Sugary smoothies** (Use unsweetened almond milk without oils—*Pure Harvest* is great. Limit fruit and stick to *one serve of fruit per day.*)
- **Heavy, creamy sauces**
- **Alcohol**
- **Cheese** (in large amounts; cottage cheese is fine)
- **Nuts** (in large handfuls because they are easy to overdo)

- **Sugary yoghurts** (stick to natural Greek yoghurt)
- **Cereal**
- **Fast food**
- **Fruit** *(limit to one low-GI serve per day):*
    - 1 apple
    - ½ banana
    - ¾ cup berries
    - ½ cup papaya/pawpaw

A Note on Bread...

You must test your commitment with this innocent-looking bystander. I have a love–hate relationship with bread. Actually, that's a lie; it's just love. I also know it doesn't love me back. I ghosted bread for the first six days of my reset, then one morning had two slices with Vegemite. Less than half an hour later, I looked four months pregnant. That swiftly ended our romance.

I'll revisit bread eventually, but not until I'm at my ideal weight, and even then, only the well-bred kind—occasionally, not as a daily indulgence.

After all, I am *not* French.
Touché.

Foods to Enjoy Freely During the 30-Day Reset:

These foods support digestion, stabilise blood sugar, reduce inflammation, and help regulate appetite. Build your meals from this list as often as you like.

Proteins

- Eggs
- Chicken breast or thigh

- Turkey
- Lean beef
- Lamb (lean cuts)
- White fish (such as barramundi, snapper and flathead; all are readily available and low in mercury)
- Salmon or tinned salmon
- Tinned tuna or sardines
- Prawns
- Firm tofu or tempeh
- Cottage cheese
- Plain Greek yoghurt (unsweetened)

Vegetables (unlimited)

Especially the ones that support digestion and reduce bloat:

- Zucchini
- Broccoli
- Bok choy
- Cabbage
- Spinach
- Rocket
- Kale
- Green beans
- Snow peas

- Carrot
- Celery
- Cucumber
- Lettuce
- Tomatoes
- Mushrooms
- Cauliflower

Healthy Fats (small amounts)

- Extra virgin olive oil, hemp seed oil or avocado oil
- Avocado (¼–½ per day)
- Chia seeds (1 tsp max)
- Flax/LSA
- Pumpkin seeds
- Sunflower seeds

Herbs, Spices + Extras

- Ginger
- Garlic
- Lemon/lime juice
- Fresh herbs
- Low-sodium soy sauce
- Vinegar (apple cider, balsamic, rice vinegar)

- Mustard
- Kimchi or sauerkraut (fermented foods support digestion)

Foods to Enjoy in Moderation:

These aren't "bad" foods, they just require portion awareness during The Reset because they impact hunger, insulin or inflammation more than people realise.

Starchy Foods (low-GI options only)

- Dense rye bread or true sourdough (max 2 thin slices/day)
- Brown rice
- Quinoa
- Low-GI potatoes (1 baby/small potato with a meal)

Fruit (1 serve per day—choose low GI)

- 1 apple
- ¾ cup berries
- ½ banana (the rest keeps fine for later)
- ½ cup papaya/pawpaw
- 1 small pear or ½ medium pear

Nuts (small portions)

- Walnuts
- Pistachios
- Hazelnuts

- Almonds
  (1 small handful = enough. They are very easy to overeat.)

Dairy

- Milk in coffee
- Small amounts of cheese
- Greek yoghurt (unsweetened but watch portions)

Sweeteners (minimal)

- Honey
- Maple syrup
- Coconut sugar
  (Use sparingly and avoid daily.)

This is your metabolic reset phase. Your maintenance phase comes later.

What Happens to Your Body When You Eat This Way:

✓ Belly deflates

✓ Face sharpens

✓ Waist shrinks

✓ Digestion smooths

✓ Hormones stabilise

✓ Insulin lowers

✓ Cravings disappear

✓ Sleep deepens

✓ Fat-burning increases

✓ Confidence rises

This is the transformation most women were never taught was possible.

In my second pregnancy, gestational diabetes was detected, strangely not in my first. This meant I could directly compare the two pregnancies, and because my daughters were born just nineteen months apart, it was a fair comparison. I had not aged dramatically or made any major lifestyle changes, other than suddenly having a new human to keep alive.

Following my diagnosis, I had to follow a carefully controlled diet for the next sixteen weeks. The food I ate was very close to what I recommend in this reset (all low GI and low GL), and the difference in how I felt and looked was remarkable. I had stable energy, gained only true baby weight, and felt far more energised in the early weeks after my second daughter was born, even while chasing a toddler around.

That said, I'm not recommending this approach for pregnant or gestating mothers without medical guidance. Pregnancy requires additional calories and nutrients, so always discuss dietary changes with your healthcare provider.

In the next chapter, we look at life on and beyond The Reset.

SIX

Drinks, Hunger And Real Life

Real life... sigh.

You will get tired in the beginning. You may get emotional. People will offer you cake, which will be hard to refuse. And on some days, you may even find yourself contemplating eating an entire loaf of bread by yourself.

So how do we navigate life without living like a stoic?

By preparing for the moments *between* the plan: cravings, stress, off days, social situations and the evenings when cooking feels too hard.

Alongside my lifelong devotion to bread, wine and I shared a long, beautiful love affair. I even co-owned a wine shop in Melbourne, which tells you everything you need to know about my commitment level.

But here's the truth: alcohol slows progress, especially belly fat loss.

During The Reset, treat alcohol like a long-distance relationship. Enjoy it occasionally and spend more time with water. Alcohol disrupts sleep, hormones, appetite and digestion and it pauses fat burning. Every time you drink, your liver deals with alcohol first, not fat metabolism.

If you can avoid alcohol altogether during The Reset, do so. If not, keep it to weekends and stick to one, perhaps two. A little French philosophy helps here: life is meant to be enjoyed, wine is enjoyable and hangovers are not, therefore enjoy wine in moderation.

Eating Out

It's not the challenge it used to be. Most places offer lighter options. Ask for sweeteners and condiments on the side.

Breakfast: eggs with mushrooms, spinach, tomato; or a simple smoothie
Lunch: protein + salad with light dressing
Dinner: protein + vegetables
Travelling: follow the same principles

If it's white, starchy, or designed to soak up sauces, skip it during The Reset. The Reset is portable; it works anywhere.

"What if I'm starving at night?"

Check your dinner timing. Most night-time hunger is timing, not true hunger.

If you genuinely need something, have herbal tea or a warm almond milk with cinnamon, two spoons of yoghurt or simply go to bed early. You are not meant to fight cravings at 11pm. You are meant to sleep.

"What if I mess up?"

You can't.

One meal doesn't undo anything. The solution is always the same: your next meal.

If you slip for a few days or even months, you haven't ruined anything. You can reset at any moment.

"What if I get bored?"

If your palate feels bored, a short water fast can help reset things, but only after you're comfortable on the plan.

A 14–18 hour fast gives the digestive system a rest and sharpens your taste for cleaner foods, and a good portion of it takes place while you sleep. If you try it, do it safely: eat a nourishing dinner beforehand, have water, black coffee and electrolytes during the fast, and break it gently with a smoothie then protein. Stop if you feel unwell.

Remember, boredom is often dopamine withdrawal. When you remove constant sugar, snacking and scrolling, calm can feel strange. Stick with it; it settles. This is a reset, not a prison.

The Three Types of Hunger

Biological hunger:

True physical hunger. Gentle hollowness, mild pangs, neutral and steady. You could eat now or later.

Habit hunger:

"I always eat now" hunger shows up as afternoon snacks, dessert after dinner, or food with coffee. This fades when you stop reinforcing it.

Emotional hunger:

Urgent and dramatic. Triggered by stress, boredom, loneliness, PMS, exhaustion, frustration, or feeling unappreciated.
This hunger seeks relief, not food.

The Real Reasons You Get Cravings

Cravings are chemistry, not character.

1. Hormone-driven cravings: low oestrogen, high cortisol, insulin spikes, PMS, perimenopause.
2. Blood sugar cravings: spike → crash → urgent cravings.
3. Gut-driven cravings: certain bacteria crave sugar or carbs—as your microbiome shifts, cravings shift.
4. Dopamine loop cravings: stress → eat, bored → eat, avoiding feelings → eat.

The Reset breaks the loop.

How to Stop Cravings Fast

1. Delay 20 minutes: most cravings fade quickly.
2. Change your state: move rooms, walk, stretch.
3. Drink something warm: herbal tea calms false hunger.
4. Remove triggers: environment beats willpower.
5. Ask: "Stomach or mouth?" If an egg sounds good, you're hungry. If only chocolate will do, you're not.
6. Breathe deeply for 30–60 seconds: this lowers cortisol.

Emotional Eating: The Real Truth

Emotional eating is nervous-system care, not a lack of discipline.

Types include:

• Stress eating
• Comfort eating
• Avoidance eating

How to Stop Emotional Eating:

1. Pause and label it: "This is emotional hunger."
2. Name the emotion: tired, overwhelmed, lonely, anxious, annoyed, resentful.
3. Opposite action: walk, message someone, tidy one drawer.
4. Delay five minutes, breathe, make tea, then decide.

Overeating and "Falling Off the Wagon"

Binges happen when you get too hungry, try to be perfect, emotions build, protein and fibre are low, alcohol lowers inhibition, hormones swing, or you're exhausted or overwhelmed.

How to Recover From a Binge

- Do not restrict
- Drink water slowly
- Eat protein at your next meal
- Go to bed early
- Do not weigh yourself
- Return to structure at the next meal (not Monday)
- There is no wagon, just your next choice

How to Prevent Binges Long-Term

- Prioritise protein and fibre
- Keep meals simple
- Avoid extreme rules
- Keep alcohol low
- Protect your sleep
- Don't let yourself get too hungry
- Eat dinner early
- Serene evenings
- Keep healthy snacks on hand

When these pieces fall into place, appetite, hormones, mood and energy stabilise. The key is to interrupt the downward spiral early. As soon as you feel yourself slipping, return to your reset.

Night-Time Eating: The Witching Hour

Evenings are the most common overeating window because tension drops, boredom rises, emotions surface, decision fatigue peaks, wine is nearby and old habits return.

The fix: early dinner, kitchen closed, early shower, warm lights, peaceful wind-down, early bedtime, avoid alcohol. A relaxed evening means fewer cravings.

The Emotional Hangover After Overeating

Guilt, shame, regret and panic are normal. But one meal doesn't undo anything. Move on.

Why This Chapter Matters

In my younger years, I believed weight loss was about exercise. Later, I thought it was about food. Eventually, I realised it is never that simple.

Our appetite and cravings are shaped by hormones, sleep, stress, emotions, habits and the nervous system, all things women are rarely taught to notice.

When you understand those signals, and simplify the way you respond to them, the whole journey becomes a lot calmer. Food and exercise matter, but they're just two pieces of a much bigger puzzle.

What You'll Notice Next

Women who tune into their hunger rhythms and eat according to their physical needs at the right times of day experience fewer cravings, fewer binges, stable eating, better sleep, fewer emotional spirals, easier weight loss and more confidence. Food stops feeling chaotic, your body feels predictable again and you finally feel in control.

Many people struggle with silence in a conversation and feel compelled to fill the gap. The same thing happens with food. A pause between meals can feel uncomfortable, as if something is missing. But it isn't a void; it's a space your body can rest in.

Allow it. Enjoy the break, the quiet, the moment where nothing is being asked of you.

SEVEN
The Reset Progress Report

Week One: The Week Everything Feels Different (In Good Ways and Weird Ways)

I have a love-hate relationship with Week One. I always start full of enthusiasm, but it ebbs and flows. Getting through that first week is the hardest part for me.

After seven days, I am suddenly much easier to negotiate with.

'You have made it this far.'

'You do not want to start again.'

'Only a few more weeks to go.'

I give myself these little pep talks just to stay on track.

Otherwise, I will be ordering a slab of Vanilla Slice to be flown in from Banana Boogie Bakery. Apparently it is the best.

Week One has a special feel of its own. It is a good week to move on from, but it is not all bad, so do not worry.

It is the week where your body is adjusting, your brain is negotiating and your subconscious knows you are up to something.

Most people expect Week One of any diet or reset to feel either magical or miserable, but the truth sits somewhere in the middle. It's a week of subtle shifts, the odd surprising moment and a few early wins, even if you cannot see them yet because they're happening quietly inside your body.

The first things most women notice are not weight loss, but the signs that the body is recalibrating. You might experience:

- diarrhoea in the early days as your body moves waste and toxins through
- flatulence as the gut begins repairing
- bloating as your fibre intake increases

None of these symptoms are pleasant and they can make you question what you have started, but they are completely normal and only temporary. They are simply signs that your system is adjusting.

By the end of Week One, many women notice:

- a spring in their step
- hunger calming down
- digestion behaving again
- bloating beginning to reduce
- a smoother-looking face, maybe even a glow
- a brain that finally stops thinking about food every 20 minutes

You may brace for hunger, panic, deprivation or drama, but when your breakfasts and lunches are simple, grounded and nutritious, your body is not running on sugar spikes. Your appetite evens out, cravings quieten and you feel stable.

That stability becomes the foundation of the entire reset.

The Quirks of Week One

There are the "is this normal?" moments, which include light-headedness, bowel movements reinventing themselves, emotions popping up out of nowhere and sudden waves of tiredness. When When I started Yeppoonie Smoothie, I had no idea I was opening up a whole world of bowel-movement conversations as customers shared every detail with zero hesitation. I would reiterate that this is simply your biology responding exactly as it should.

Everything is adjusting:

- your gut
- your hormones
- your stress response
- your blood sugar
- your evening habits
- your sleep
- your energy (less jittery, more grounded)

Most women hit Day 4 or 5 and wake up thinking, "Something is different." They cannot always describe it, they just feel lighter, calmer, less puffy, more themselves. That is not weight loss yet. It is inflammation stepping aside, announcing the very first whisper of The Reveal Phase.

The Emotional Declutter

Another classic Week One moment is emotional clarity. When you are not eating chaotically, your feelings have nowhere to hide.

You start seeing:

- your cravings for what they really are
- which habits were autopilot
- which thoughts were stress-driven
- how much "evening hunger" was in fact emotional hunger

I expected Week One to be a battle, but once I worked out the ideal portion sizes, the right snacking moments, the foods that suited me and increased my water intake, I settled into a steady rhythm. By the end of the week, I was not thinking about food nearly as much, which is half the battle. I would make enough dinner to last two nights, and because I was limiting my dinner to protein and vegetables, I simply bought eggs, chicken, one beef steak, a packet of tofu and a variety of vegetables I knew I would use. I shopped less and spent less. Win-win.

You will also find that:

- your body starts trusting you again
- your hunger becomes predictable
- your stomach stops sabotaging you
- your clothes begin sitting differently, even slightly (my favourite part)
- you feel lighter and pain-free without the niggling inflammation

Timelines and Quirks: Why Everyone Responds Differently

It is worth noting that time frames for symptoms, signs and weight loss vary from person to person. Your week-one effects might not show up until week two, and vice versa.

If you are hungry all the time and feel unprepared, your mind will naturally fixate on food. That is why staying well-nourished is essential while you adjust to foods you may not be used to eating and withdraw from the ones you relied on before. Bread, cereals, potatoes and muffins are common break-ups, and letting them go can feel surprisingly emotional. A fridge full of goodness and simple snacks makes all the difference.

Stick with it. As your microbiome improves with extra fibre and nutrients, cravings for old favourites, especially the sweet treats that certain gut bacteria feed on begin to fade. Before long, you will genuinely enjoy fresh, healthy food every day.

The Week One Realisation

By the end of Week One, you start to realise you can actually do this. And it is. If you can get through Week One, which is arguably the hardest, Week Two will feel like a breeze.

EIGHT

The Reveal Phase: When Everything Finally Starts to Shift

Waking up one morning and feeling lighter, seeing a flatter stomach, a softer waistline, a face that looks more rested, is the moment you realise it's not some impossible fantasy. It's not something that only happens to other people, the ones with perfect discipline or a private chef. If you stick to The Reset and settle into the rhythm, it becomes inevitable: your body will finally let you see the progress it's been quietly working on behind the scenes.

Most women don't gain weight the way they think they do. What actually happens is that the body gradually becomes inflamed, stressed, under-slept and overwhelmed. Digestion slows down, hormones become jumpy and fluid retention builds up. All of that sits on top of your actual body like a puffy layer of noise. It looks like fat. It feels like fat. But it isn't quite fat, not yet.

The Reveal Phase is the moment that layer finally dissolves.

It's not magic and fat cells don't miraculously vanish overnight. What's really happening is far more logical: your digestion settles, inflammation drops, your hormones stop fluctuating wildly, your appetite steadies and your body finally understands that your eating pattern is predictable. When all of that lines up, your shape changes quickly, often in a surprising way because it feels sudden, even though it isn't.

Most people experience their first Reveal Phase around the end of the first week or sometime in the second. Some feel it earlier, especially if they've been bloated or inflamed for a long time. For others it takes a little longer. The moment is unmistakable, though. You wake up and your stomach feels noticeably flatter. Clothes that felt tight a few days ago suddenly slip on without resistance. Your face looks more defined. You feel lighter walking around the house. Hunger feels regulated, cravings quieter and your whole system just seems... easier.

Many women say it feels like their body has deflated overnight, not in a dramatic way, but enough to be noticeable. You might realise that your rings fit better, your waist feels softer, or the waistband on your jeans doesn't leave a mark anymore. You feel different internally too; something inside you releases, like your body has finally exhaled after holding its breath for months. You may even notice you're breathing more easily.

And here's the important part: when you reach this moment, you don't need to change anything. In fact, the only mistake women make during the Reveal Phase is assuming it's a sign they can relax the plan. They'll add extra snacks, pour a cheeky wine or three, eat a bigger dinner or add more ingredients to meals "since things are going well." It's human nature to assume the hard part is over.

Remember, your body is just beginning to trust the new rhythm, so the best thing you can do is stay consistent. Keep your meals simple, drink water and stick to earlier dinners. Do not rush ahead and do not sabotage yourself by trying to "reward" the progress.

Once you hold your structure for a few more days, the Reveal Phase deepens. It comes in waves. You'll have days where you feel dramatically better, followed by days where things feel slower. That's normal. The body doesn't release everything in one dramatic sweep; it does it layer by layer. Release, stabilise, release, stabilise. Each wave feels easier than the last.

Another thing I noticed personally, is that fat loss comes in weird stages. Of course it didn't happen in the order I wanted it to. It tends to follow this pattern, the "outer" areas tend to lean out first, while the deep, hormonally active fat around the belly is always the last to shift. Naturally, it's the very area we want to shrink first, which feels like yet another slightly unfair mystery of being a woman.

You may notice your face, collarbones, arms and even your upper back looking slimmer before your waistline budges at all. Then the hips, thighs and lower body slowly begin to change. It will not happen all at once, but it will happen.

Then this strange thing occurs, which I now call the "jelly stage."

About a week or so in, I caught my reflection one morning and thought I looked worse than when I started. Not bigger, just... odd. Softer. Looser. Almost unflattering in a way I did not expect. My first thought was, *I am never wearing a bikini again.* Now I fully understand where the term "jelly belly" comes from.

But there's a very normal explanation: the firm outer layer of fat begins to soften first, and the deeper, more stubborn layers are loosening underneath. It's a transition phase, like a wave pulling back before it rolls forward.

Expect to look slightly worse before you look better. It's simply your body shifting and preparing for the real reveal to come.

This stage is actually one of the clearest signs, the proof you've been looking for, that things are moving in the right direction. Progress: jelly-like, wobbly, not very glamorous... but progress all the same.

If you stay consistent through this stage, the shape comes. It always does. The jelly phase doesn't last forever, but almost every woman goes through it, including me. And the more you understand what's happening inside your body, the less likely you are to panic and the more likely you are to see the real change arrive.

Emotions

When you've been feeling stuck or frustrated for months and then suddenly feel hopeful again, a deep sense of peace comes over you, a quiet knowing that everything will be okay. The inner critic is hushed, you stop worrying that something is wrong with your health, and you learn to trust both the process and your ability to follow through. You feel in control of your well-being. It's a quiet confidence that becomes fuel to keep going.

I also found myself much calmer when dealing with stressful situations; things that annoyed me a month earlier suddenly passed over me like water off a duck's back. Minor irritations with people and situations just...went away. I even felt more patient at long traffic lights, not that I was a road-rager before.

This unexpected evolution was a pleasant and rewarding bonus. I hoped more such surprises were still to come.

The Reveal Phase is not an ending; it is the beginning. It is the moment that proves your body is responsive, not resistant. It is where you realise that the simplicity of the plan is not boring, it is brilliant. And it is the point where your body shows you what it is capable of once it is no longer drowning in confusion and stress.

NINE

The Middle Weeks: Where the Real Change Happens

Human nature is such that the excitement of starting something new always fades. The first week of The Reset feels fresh, purposeful and for some even fun. You are making moves, your meals are clear, you are patting yourself on the back and your motivation is practically humming.

But it is the middle weeks, the second, third, and sometimes the early part of the fourth, that determine whether this reset becomes a success or just another attempt you quietly abandon.

For me, Week Three, on a Friday no less, is where things got a bit wobbly. Not just physically, but psychologically. Not because The Reset was difficult, but because this is the stage where old habits try to negotiate their way back in. Suddenly I found myself thinking about bread again, and then wine began whispering my name from the fridge. It felt a little biblical, like my own miniature "forty days in the desert" moment. The temptation was real.

I did not want to foil my plan, which was unfolding beautifully, and I could see that meaningful transformation was already happening. So I did not give in. I went for a walk, and the temptation passed as quickly and quietly as it arrived. I knew it was just a moment inside a phase. Your brain simply needs time to adjust to the new rhythm until it finally cements itself.

It is a bit like making sourdough bread: it starts soft, it needs shaping, and it only becomes something solid with consistency and time.

It is also helpful to remember that your mind will get restless long before your body is finished transforming. Your body is quietly doing its job, while your mind is bored senseless and looking elsewhere for entertainment.

What is actually happening physically?

During the middle weeks, digestion becomes increasingly efficient and energy starts to smooth out. Inflammation drops, cravings lose their power, and sleep noticeably improves. Your stomach feels more predictable from day to day, and your appetite stabilises so much that you stop thinking about food as often. Even your face and waistline shift subtly, and clothes that felt tight only weeks earlier begin to sit more comfortably.

Some days it does not feel noticeable at all, which is exactly why consistency matters.

Like your bank account, so they say, your body does its best work when you are not paying attention. So do not assume a quiet day means nothing is happening. I like to think the "nothing to report" days are the ones creating the deepest changes, the interest quietly accruing.

And keep in mind that there is a part of your subconscious that absolutely dislikes change. It feels uncomfortable, unfamiliar and a little threatening, so it tries to pull you back to your old patterns, the ones that did not serve you well but felt safe simply because you lived in them for so long. Your subconscious is not trying to sabotage you; it just prefers what it recognises, even if that was not good for you.

I find that a bit scary, because it suggests I really am my own worst enemy. Oh wait... I am.

The only way through is to believe, wholeheartedly and unapologetically, that you are better off now than you were before you started. Do not romanticise the old version of you; do not even look back.

Take it one day at a time but keep your eye firmly on the prize. That alone snaps the subconscious into line.

The key in the middle weeks is to trust the new rhythm you have created. There is no need to rush ahead, add extra rules, or start complicating things just to keep it interesting. Keeping it simple is what allows your body to settle and do the work.

If you feel tempted or restless, change your scenery rather than your food. Go for a walk, phone a friend, clean a drawer, or even an entire room; by the end of the month your home will be noticeably tidier, one small corner at a time. Choose anything that occupies your mind but still allows your body to stay in the routine that is helping you progress.

And remember this: every woman who completes a 30-day reset eventually looks back and realises that the breakthrough happened in the middle weeks of this marathon. It does not happen in the first week, when motivation is high and everything feels new. It does not happen in the final week, when momentum carries you forward almost automatically. It happens in the middle, when you choose ongoing commitment instead of excitement, and that choice changes everything.

As any turtle knows, slow and steady wins the race, or in this case, slow and steady transforms your body.

In the next chapter, we will talk about what to do when progress slows down, how to recognise the difference between a plateau and a pause, and why the body does not work in a straight line (even when your mind really wishes it would).

TEN

When Progress Slows: And Why That's Usually the Best Sign of All

Every woman who has ever tried to improve her health knows the feeling: the early progress arrives, you feel lighter, you feel proud, your clothes start cooperating again... and then out of nowhere, everything seems to pause. Not go backwards, just stop. As if your body has suddenly gone on strike.

This is the point where most women panic. They assume their body has "adjusted" and that they need to shake things up, do more, eat less, tighten the plan, ramp everything to the extreme.

And suddenly the questions start spiralling:

Is this even working?
Is something wrong?
Is my body being difficult again?
Did I break it?
Was that one snack three days ago the beginning of the end?
Should I start exercising more?

This is the mental storm that hits right before the next breakthrough, and exactly when you need to do the opposite of what your panic is telling you.

Women have been conditioned to interpret a pause as failure, when in reality a pause is simply part of the process. Bodies don't change like a straight line on a graph, they change in a series of steps. Progress, in the real world, is rarely linear. It moves, stabilises, moves again, takes a breath, and continues.

Your body isn't stalling because it's stubborn.
It's pausing because it's recalibrating.

A pause is often the moment your body is rearranging itself internally, shifting hormones, balancing fluid, improving digestion, repairing gut lining, reducing inflammation, adjusting appetite signals, and deciding what comes next. It's incredibly busy inside even when it looks uneventful outside. Remember, the human body is amazing.

This is why the middle stretch can feel confusing. You feel better, but you don't necessarily feel lighter every single day. Your stomach may be flat some mornings and a little rounder the next. Your energy may be consistent one week and patchy the next. Your face may look more defined one day and softer the next. None of this is regression, it's ebb and flow.

Think of it like the tide.
It comes in, then it pulls back.
It never retreats because something went wrong; it's simply following a rhythm.
Your body works the same way.

And here's the beautiful thing: the women who resist the urge to panic during the pauses, who hold steady and trust the method instead of scrambling for a quick fix, are the women who experience the deepest Reveal Phases later.

The body rewards consistency, not anxiety.

If you push harder, your body tightens.
If you panic, it holds on.
If you start cutting meals or skipping food, it becomes more protective.

But if you stay stable, keep your meals balanced, drink your smoothies, have your simple dinners, and give your system predictability, your body begins to relax again. And when it relaxes, it lets go. Remember the principle I learned from the midwife: open mind, open body. When your thoughts are clearer and the routine feels predictable, your body follows that lead and releases what it has been holding onto.

In my experience, the biggest visible progress always happens after a slow stretch. I'll go through several quiet days with no noticeable change, and then suddenly wake up feeling lighter, more defined, and my skirt that wouldn't zip last week suddenly zips up with ease.

It feels like "out of nowhere," but nothing in the body happens out of nowhere. It happened because no one interfered with the quiet work happening beneath the surface.

I knew to expect this because I was aware of the concept of plateaus. Many people misunderstand the idea of "plateaus." A true plateau during a 30-day reset is rare. More often, people are experiencing one of two things: either their body is resting and integrating the progress, or their mind is getting impatient and projecting frustration onto a perfectly normal process. Most of the time, it's the second one.

You don't need to overhaul anything during these moments. You don't need to eat less, move more, punish yourself, or create tighter rules. The plan doesn't need to be more extreme; it needs to be consistent. Just like in the previous chapter, these are common battles in the middle weeks of the 30-day reset.

If you stay consistent here, everything becomes easier. If you hold your rhythm, the Reveal Phase returns. And when it returns, it often makes up for every moment you doubted yourself.

In the next chapter, we'll explore the emotional side of transformation, the surprising ways your identity shifts when your body finally catches up to the version of yourself you've always known was there.

ELEVEN

When Your Body Changes, Your Identity Shifts Too

One of the strangest things about transforming your body, especially after years of feeling stuck, is how emotional it can be. People talk endlessly about weight loss in terms of food, discipline, steps, macros, calories, motivation... but almost no one talks about the identity shift that happens when you finally start feeling like yourself again.

It starts subtly. One morning you wake up and feel a bit clearer. As you get dressed, you notice your jeans are no longer cutting you in half. You catch your reflection and see the real you again, not a younger version, but the you who feels grounded, clear, and comfortable in your own skin. You move differently in your kitchen, and you walk with lighter steps. You feel more in control of your day, as if a weight you did not even realise you were carrying has quietly slipped off your shoulders.

When you have felt heavy, bloated, foggy or inflamed for a long time, that feeling becomes part of your identity. You do not do it consciously, it just happens. You start seeing yourself as the woman who is always tired, always dragging herself around, always trying to fix herself but never quite getting there. You get used to feeling puffy, achy or off. Your clothes stop sitting right, you avoid photos and you ignore your own discomfort because there is no time to unpack it.

So when your body begins to shift and that heaviness lifts, it does something strange to your mind. It wakes you up. You start paying attention, and you start believing change is possible after all. Your shoulders sit differently, you expect more from your day, and you engage with the world and those in it in ways you have not in a long time. You begin making decisions from clarity rather than fatigue. It feels as if someone has taken a dimmer switch and slowly turned the lights back on.

There is a moment that often arrives in the middle of your reset when you realise you have not boiled your usual potatoes or prepared rice for quite some time, and you do not miss them. You make your coffee and notice you no longer reach automatically for the sugar, and you pause, realising you do not need it. It lands with a quiet sense of pride: *I am doing this. I am actually doing it.* You shift from trying to being, from hoping to trusting, from doubting to knowing. Once that shift happens, everything becomes easier and things begin to flow.

Food becomes less emotional and alcohol loses its power. Evenings feel calmer and mornings feel clearer. Your self-image starts to update itself to match your behaviour instead of your past, and your habits strengthen because your identity is finally catching up. You stop feeling like someone who is trying to lose weight and start feeling like someone who simply takes care of herself.

This is why women who complete a reset often say the physical changes were only half of the transformation. The deeper shift was in how they saw themselves, how they moved through the world, how they spoke to themselves with more kindness, and how they made decisions with more clarity.

You notice you are no longer feeling ashamed or behind. You notice you are not dragging the old version of yourself around like a shadow. The Reset changes your body, and consistency changes your habits, but identity is what changes your life. That, more than anything, is why this reset works. It allows women to reconnect with the part of themselves they thought they had lost.

TWELVE

Movement: Why Gentle Wins

If there's one area where women have been spectacularly misled, it's exercise. Somewhere along the way, movement stopped being something that supported our bodies and turned into something we were supposed to survive. Boot camps, 5am HIIT sessions, kettlebells being flung around like weapons...it is no wonder women feel exhausted.

And women, being women, took the assignment seriously.
We tried to be warriors.
We tried to keep up.
We tried to convince ourselves that collapsing on the floor after a workout was a badge of honour rather than a clear sign our nervous systems had left the chat.

But our bodies have been telling us the truth for years: the older we get, the worse we respond to punishing workouts. What might have "worked" in our twenties, and by worked, I mostly mean made us sweaty and hungry, simply doesn't serve us now. Not hormonally, not emotionally, not physically.

With age, the body begins to work differently. Recovery takes longer, sleep becomes lighter, energy fluctuates, and hormones become more sensitive to stress. It is not a sign that anything is wrong, only that your body is asking for a gentler approach.

Women contact us at Yeppoonie Smoothie saying the same thing: "I'm doing everything right, I'm hitting the gym harder, but I feel and look worse. I'm making no progress."

There's a reason for this.

The female body does not thrive under constant stress.
It doesn't like being pushed into the red zone every day.

I have, as a guinea-pig person, been through both extremes many times. And what I learned is that getting my diet in order far surpassed exercise alone, or even exercise paired with half-hearted diet improvement.

When women shift to gentler movement, the kind that lifts the heart rate without frying the nervous system, everything begins to settle. Hunger becomes predictable. Cravings drop away. Evenings feel calmer. Sleep deepens. The body does not panic from the effort; it absorbs it.

Walking is the perfect example.

It looks unimpressive, but it quietly does what brutal workouts do not: it steadies you. A fast walk clears your head, regulates cortisol, warms the body without inflaming it, and leaves you feeling lighter instead of depleted. It is the kind of movement you can do every day without planning your whole life around recovery.

The same goes for Pilates, yoga, gentle strength training, swimming, and slow cycling, all of which support you rather than punish you. They create tone and energy instead of hunger and exhaustion. They help you build a strong body without feeling like you are auditioning for an episode of *Survivor*.

A walk every day will do more for your body than five frantic workouts you dread. Strength training done consistently will reshape you faster than any bootcamp ever could.

When you stop using movement to "fix" yourself and start using it to care for yourself, everything changes. You no longer drag your body to workouts out of guilt. You move because it feels good, because it lifts your mood, clears your mind, and reminds you that you are not here to punish yourself into becoming smaller.

You are here to live in a body that feels serene, capable, strong and grounded.

In the next chapter, we move into a topic women underestimate until they fix it: sleep. It's where the dream body, the predictable appetite, the good mood and the flatter stomach often begin.

THIRTEEN

Sleep: The Silent Factor That Changes Everything

There's a reason sleep is the first thing to fall apart when life gets stressful, and the last thing to repair itself when you finally start taking care of yourself again. Women underestimate the influence of sleep on their bodies more than almost anything else. We treat it like a luxury, not a foundation. But if your sleep is out of order, everything else will be too.

Your evening impacts your morning.

You may have noticed: if you go to bed angry or miserable, you wake up feeling the same way. That's why developing, and embracing, a calm, simple evening rhythm matters more than most women realise.

You can eat well, drink water, take supplements, walk every day, meditate, journal, go to therapy, and buy a fancy pillow spray full of empty promises, but if you're not sleeping properly, your body will quietly protest. It will keep you inflamed, hungry, irritable and slightly off-balance.

Women feel the effects of poor sleep more intensely because our hormones are sensitive creatures. A single night of interrupted or shallow rest can throw off your appetite the next day. It can make cravings louder. It can make your stomach puffier. It can make stress feel bigger than it actually is. It can turn a small emotional wobble into a full-blown spiral.

And ironically, women often sleep poorly for reasons they no longer even notice: rushing, overstimulation (hello, Netflix), alcohol, emotional load, scrolling, late-night eating, late-night thinking, late-night everything.

We collapse into bed exhausted, but because we are wired from the overstimulation of the day and evening, we wake up feeling no better. We do not feel replenished at all; the tank is still empty.

We assume this is just what adulthood feels like.

The Reset improves sleep without you deliberately targeting it. Early dinner, smooth digestion, stable blood sugar, and a settled appetite all create the internal conditions your body needs to unwind. These signals quietly tell your nervous system:

"It's safe to power down now."

It is not about consciously controlling anything; it is about giving your body the environment it needs so it can finally do what it has been trying to do all along at night: rest, repair and reset.

Women often tell me they have not slept this well in years after starting the Yeppoonie Smoothie Good Evening blend. It is not because they changed as sleepers, but because they finally stopped over-stressing their bodies and created a peaceful evening rhythm.

By the second week, you often notice that sleep begins to change its texture. It feels deeper, you fall asleep faster and you wake clearer. Your dreams feel less chaotic and your mornings less foggy. You no longer wake up feeling as if your soul left your body during the night. It is subtle but profound. A well-rested woman is calmer and less reactive. Her cravings quieten, her digestion smooths, her weight responds and her appearance brightens. Her eyes look clearer, lighter and more alive.

When sleep improves, everything becomes easier, even the psychological elements. You cope better. You think straight. You make better food decisions because your brain actually has the capacity to make them. You're not leaning on sugar, carbs, or alcohol just to stay upright.

Sleep lets your body do the repair work it simply cannot do while you're awake. That's why you can't fix food problems with food alone, because so many of them actually begin with sleep. We need to love our beds in the evening as much as we do in the morning, when we're in no hurry to leave them.

One thing that has improved my own sleep is turning my bedroom into a little sanctuary. When your space feels calm and welcoming, you genuinely want to get to bed earlier. It nourishes you in the same way a bowl of homemade soup does on a cold day.

I remember as a teenager that it was crucial my bedroom felt like my own space, despite the unfortunate pink velvet curtains and floral wallpaper eight-year-old me had chosen (proof that children should not be given décor autonomy). Still, I made it cosy and I slept like a champion. Of course, back then there was no scrolling, just turning the pages of a book, the perfect entrée to sleep.

So...tidy your space.
Organise your clothes.
Declutter.
Dust.
Open the windows and air it out.
Keep the room fresh and pleasant to be in.

You don't need to rush out and invest in expensive linen.
The magic is in the order and the cleanliness. As they say, cleanliness is next to godliness.

FOURTEEN

The Emotional Load: The Weight Women Carry That No One Sees

Every woman carries two kinds of weight: the weight on her body and the weight on her mind. The second often feels heavier.

It truly is a blessing and a curse being a woman. When you cross 40, the same pressure you took in your stride at 30 can suddenly knock the wind out of you at 45. Cortisol fires up faster and cools down slower. Progesterone, your natural calmer, starts drifting away just when you really, *really* need it. Oestrogen swinging like a pendulum is anything but soothing. Layer that with kids, work, ageing parents, relationships, hot flushes and the joy of training a learner driver, and of course you feel wrung out. Your body isn't malfunctioning, it's responding exactly as any woman's would under that kind of load. And for me personally, the overlap between menopause and raising teenage girls felt like my own teenage karma returning for a sequel.

It's exhausting, it feels endless, and it leaks into everything, especially food. Women blame their discipline, thinking they're weak or inconsistent. But discipline isn't the problem. It's depletion.

When you're carrying too much emotionally, your body looks for relief anywhere it can find it. Food (and alcohol or Netflix) becomes the quiet place you don't have anywhere else, the single moment of comfort in a day where everyone else has taken a slice of you.

That's why "just eat better" never works. It ignores the real problem: you're running on fumes. When you're inwardly spent, you don't simply crave food, you crave a break. You crave distraction. You crave something that takes the edge off.

When I made the decision to slow down my life and simplify everything, from my household to my business, the load that lifted was enormous. From that point, everything started to flow. I also felt a lot more at peace.

That's why this reset feels so different from others. Not because the food is special, but because the structure reduces emotional friction. When your meals are predictable, your body stops bracing. When your day has rhythm, your mind stops spinning. When your dinner is early and simple, your evenings feel more peaceful. The daily pressures don't disappear, but they stop dictating your appetite.

When you stop overwhelming your body with constant, complicated food decisions, it becomes easier to cope with the real burdens in your life. You're not juggling everything blindly; you're anchored.

And once your appetite quiets down, you finally see just how much you've been carrying. It's confronting at first. You realise how tired you really are, how much has been on your plate, and how little space you've had for yourself. But it's also the moment things begin to shift.

FIFTEEN

The Identity Shift: When You Become...You!

One of the most surprising things was the quiet realisation that I'd become a different version of myself. I wasn't a guinea pig anymore. I actually felt human again. (I couldn't resist that one.)

And honestly, it didn't take anything dramatic. No 5am boot camps. No 12-step meal plans. No spiritual awakenings on a mountain. It was simply slowing down, following an uncomplicated way of eating, and trusting the universe, kidding, trusting my own body to do the job it was born to do.

There was no dramatic makeover, although several new wardrobe staples did make an appearance.

And there was no "new year, new me" declaration on Facebook either. There never is. Most years I'm too busy recovering from New Year's Eve, waking at 11am and waiting for the blessed moment when a hair-of-the-dog drink becomes socially acceptable again. Okay, that's me pretending I'm actually up past 10pm on New Year's Eve these days.

Women often believe identity shifts come from effort, from discipline, motivation, or willpower. But real identity shifts happen when your daily habits finally make sense for your life. When eating simply feels easier than overeating. When stopping at one coffee feels natural instead of heroic. When early dinners aren't a punishment, they're a relief.

There is a moment when you realise you're not negotiating with yourself all day. You're simply in an easy rhythm... and that moment is gold.

We're so used to constant highs and lows, hormones, emotions, food decisions, exhaustion, that we almost don't trust feeling balanced. But balance is the beginning of identity change.

You realise you're becoming the woman you once believed only willpower could create, but willpower was never part of it. It happened because you found rhythm, embraced simplicity and invited calm back in. Those three things do more than any strict plan or burst of motivation ever could.

Women often believe change requires suffering. But the strongest version of you doesn't come from force. She appears when life finally becomes still.

And in that stillness, something shifts.

You start choosing based on how you want to *feel*, not how you want to look. You stop reaching for food to take the edge off. You stop wandering into the kitchen at night out of habit. You stop searching the fridge or pantry for answers they can't give. You honour yourself in quiet, dignified ways, and those small choices build a new identity.

That's the shift.

You don't announce that you're trying to be healthy now. You don't declare a new identity. It simply becomes, *"This is just what I do."* It's a quiet dignity you carry, and it feels light.

Without you noticing, new habits stop feeling like a diet and simply become your new normal. Your body starts cooperating and your mind starts collaborating. And your internal confidence grows quietly in the background.

You know you're capable, and you can trust yourself with food. Cravings settle down, hunger feels manageable, and the worry about regaining weight eases. In its place grows a quiet ease, the kind that comes from feeling at home in your own body.

And once that happens, everything else feels lighter too. You're not thinking about dieting. You're not constantly "starting again on Monday." You're not obsessing over food or chasing motivation. You're simply living, and that, ironically, is what keeps the weight off.

The whole point of this reset isn't to turn you into a new person; it's to bring you back to the woman you were before stress, hormones, kids, life and chaos pulled you away from yourself. As Derek Walcott wrote in his moving poem *Love After Love*:

"You will greet yourself arriving
at your own door..."

In the next chapter, we'll build a long-term rhythm that feels sustainable.

SIXTEEN

Finishing Strong: The Last Stretch of the 30 Days

There's something satisfying about reaching the final part of a reset. Even if you haven't done it perfectly, no one ever does, you can feel that you've crossed a line you didn't think you'd cross. You've shown up. You've stayed on track. You've pushed through the days that felt slow, the days that felt easy, and the days when you would've happily traded your children for a dozen hot, glazed Krispy Kremes. You've proved to yourself that you're consistent, reliable and far stronger than you gave yourself credit for.

And now you are here: the home stretch. Many assume that after a long break from their usual routines, the final days of a reset will be the hardest, as if they will be desperate to return to their old ways. In reality, they are usually the calmest. You are not wrestling with cravings anymore. Your stomach is not unpredictable. Your energy is not up and down. Your appetite has settled into a reliable rhythm. Your confidence has quietly crept back. Evenings do not unravel the way they used to. And you have become surprisingly content with the simplicity of your meals. If anything, the final days feel like proof that you really can live this way, maybe not with this exact structure forever but certainly with your own version of it.

This stage is also where you realise how much time and mental space you've freed up. When you're not constantly thinking about food, sugar, bloating, clothes that don't fit, tomorrow's damage control, or what you'll "start again on Monday," you suddenly have energy for things that sat untouched for years. Little tasks get done. Or big tasks, like writing a reset book. Walks become easier. You sit differently in your own home. Even conversations feel lighter because you're not carrying the same internal noise.

So the question becomes: what now?

How do you finish strong without sprinting toward the end like a woman who's been trapped in a retreat with no snacks?

The answer is surprisingly ordinary: you just keep going exactly as you have been. No refining, no last-minute pushing, no dramatic measures to try to get "one more big drop" before day thirty. The body doesn't work like that; the last-minute push usually backfires anyway, leaving you bloated and discouraged. What your body responds to now is the same thing it has responded to all month: rhythm.

The last stretch is not for punishing yourself; it's for landing gently.
When you finish calmly, you transition calmly.
And that is the secret to not rebounding.

Another thing you may notice in this stage is that your cravings return briefly. not because your body wants sugar, but because your mind is preparing for change. It's a bit like finishing school before the holidays. You're not hungry; you're anticipating freedom. Don't take it personally. Don't interpret it as a failure. It's just psychology doing what psychology does.

If those cravings pop up, let them pass. They always do. Your body doesn't need anything extra right now. The finish line is not the time to celebrate with the very habits you've spent a month stepping out of. The celebration is already happening: in your clothes, in your energy, in your mood, in the way you carry yourself.

Finishing strong isn't about discipline; you've already proven you have that. It's about respect. Respect for the work you've done, respect for your body's effort, and respect for the version of yourself who showed up even on the days you didn't feel like it. At the end of your reset, you may feel a little emotional. You should feel proud, probably relieved, a bit taller, a little more in charge and also reflective. You've proved something to yourself, and truly: well done, you.

This is why, as we move toward the next chapter, the focus shifts from "finishing" to "continuing." The next phase isn't about staying strict forever, absolutely not, but it *is* about settling into a rhythm that keeps you feeling good without slipping back into old patterns.

It's not about being perfect. It never was, and no one is. It's about being consistent enough to keep feeling like yourself. I call it *the rhythm of flexible consistency*: a way of eating that is calm and relaxed enough for your body to trust, but flexible enough for you to actually live your life.

In the next chapter, we will move into exactly that: how to transition out of The Reset without undoing your progress, how to find your maintenance rhythm and how to carry this lighter, steadier version of yourself into everyday life without the drama, pressure or diet mentality that derails so many women.

SEVENTEEN

How To Know When You're Ready For Maintenance

Maintenance is the stage that comes after the stricter days of The Reset. It is the period where you maintain your weight loss long term. If you still have weight to lose, you may move between The Reset rhythm and the maintenance rhythm as needed. For example, you might follow four reset days and three maintenance days per week, or whatever combination feels right for your body.

You're ready for maintenance when your body and mind have truly settled, rather than just being "over it."

You're ready if:

- You've completed 30–40 days of The Reset, or
- You've reached your ideal (or close-to-ideal) weight. Healthy weight loss takes time, so this could be a month away or a year away. It depends on your starting point and your consistency.
- You feel leaner, calmer and in control
- Cravings are almost non-existent
- Your sleep has improved
- Your hunger feels predictable and stable
- You feel emotionally regulated rather than reactive

- You actually like what you see in the mirror

Here's the important part:

Don't rush into maintenance.
Give yourself the full 30–40 days.

Why?
Because this timeframe resets the systems that actually create long-term stability:

- cortisol
- insulin
- hunger hormones (ghrelin and leptin)
- oestrogen sensitivity
- sleep patterns
- liver function
- digestion
- cravings
- emotional habits
- your identity around food

This is what prevents rebound.
This is what makes the results stick.

Maintenance only works when the foundation is solid.
Give your body the time it needs.

EIGHTEEN

Your First Two Weeks of Maintenance: Exactly What to Do, Eat and Expect

The first two weeks of maintenance are the most important part of the entire journey. Not because they're difficult, they're actually quite relaxed, but because this is when your body decides whether it will hold your results or let them slip. Think of these two weeks as the "settling period." Your body has just spent a month doing deep internal rebalancing. Now it needs consistency. Don't assume maintenance means loosening the reins immediately.

Not yet.

Maintenance is not "back to normal."

Maintenance is creating your new normal.

What to Expect in the First Two Weeks

I kept wanting to call this section *What to Expect When You're Expecting... Food*, which tells you how ingrained that pregnancy book is in my brain.

• **Your hunger will feel different**

You'll feel stable, not ravenous. This is good. It means your hormones are balanced and your appetite cues are clearer.

- **Your energy will stay balanced**

No wild spikes, no sudden crashes, no frantic afternoon need for coffee or sugar.

- **Your digestion will stay smooth**

Because you're not throwing heavy, inflammatory foods back in.

- **Your cravings remain quiet**

Unless you shock your system, so let's not.

- **Your weight might shift a little**

A 200g to 700g fluctuation is normal. Anything more usually means you reintroduced foods too quickly.

Exactly What to Keep the Same (for at least two weeks)

- Breakfast and lunch structure

  (protein + fibre + slow carbs, or your smoothie)
- Early, simple dinner

  (your single biggest maintenance tool)
- One coffee, maybe two, but don't return to four
- Daily walking
- Keep alcohol out

  Your liver is stabilizing; give it time. If you must reintroduce it, wait as long as you can.
- Keep your portions predictable

  Predictability signals safety to the brain.
- Avoid night-time eating

  These two weeks are about holding your lane, not sprinting into a new one.

What You Can Gently Reintroduce

Week One of Maintenance

- A little more fruit
- A little more healthy fat
- Slightly larger lunch or dinner portions
- More variety in protein and fibre
- A second coffee occasionally (not daily)

Week Two of Maintenance

- A slice of good-quality sourdough or low-GI toast
- A small portion of whole grains
  (quinoa, brown rice, low-GI potato)
- A simple dessert once or twice if you want it
- Social meals: choose simple over rich or dramatic

If anything triggers bloating, cravings, or a spike in hunger, scale back. It's just your body communicating. This is good. Now you listen.

What to Avoid for Two Weeks

(Not forever—just while the foundation sets)

- heavy breads
- pastries
- fried food
- sweetened drinks
- huge servings of pasta
- nightly desserts
- wine/snacks on autopilot
- "cheat meals": they're just unhealthy meals and the only person you're cheating is yourself

Remember: nothing is off-limits forever.
But reintroducing everything at once is the fastest way to undo your progress.

Your Maintenance Plate (simple and dependable)

Breakfast

- Your smoothie
- OR eggs with vegetables
- OR oats + yoghurt + berries + nuts

Lunch

- Protein + vegetables + healthy fat
  (chicken bowl, tuna salad, tofu stir-fry, leftover protein + greens)

Snack *(only if hungry)*

- Handful of nuts
- Piece of fruit
- A yoghurt
- Herbal tea

Dinner

- Simple, early protein + vegetables
  (keep this exact structure for two weeks—it's magic)

Hydration

- Water or herbal tea
- Coffee earlier in the day
- Nothing stimulating at night

What Not to Worry About

- Small weight fluctuations
- Feeling slightly hungrier one day
- Mild bloating when reintroducing a food
- Eating out once
- A tired day
- A less-than-perfect day

When You'll Know It's Working

- Food no longer takes up mental space
- Hunger is predictable
- Your weight stays stable
- Evenings feel easy
- You feel "normal" rather than "in a program"
- Your clothes still fit perfectly
- You feel like yourself

Congratulations. The Reset changed you and you may even continue living this way indefinitely.

NINETEEN

Life After The Reset: Keeping the Calm Without Keeping the Rules

Life after The Reset is where you learn how to stay there. Most women can follow a new structure for a few weeks; the real challenge is what happens when the structure fades and you're back in your normal rhythm. School runs. Work. Social life. Stress. Travel. Hormones. A bad night's sleep. A birthday. A long lunch. A wine night. A flight. A heavy day. A whatever day. The list is endless.

Life never stops, but what does change is how you respond, and your response is completely within your control.

After The Reset, there's a quiet internal shift where you realise you're not scared of food, hunger, or slipping. Hold onto this. You don't need to be perfect; you simply keep hold of the threads of stability The Reset has given you and weave them into the tapestry of your real life.

Stability doesn't look like weighing lettuce or logging every crumb. It looks like noticing when you feel off, puffy, overwhelmed, hungry, or flat, and gently bringing yourself back to equilibrium. We spend so much time offering kindness to others that we forget to extend it to ourselves.

There's no panic now, no spiralling, no "stuff it, I've ruined everything." Just a calm response.

Your appetite shifts too. Heavy meals weigh you down, and rich food becomes less desirable. You might still order the pasta, but you don't feel compelled to finish the entire bowl. You stop because you're done, not because you're being "good."

Alcohol becomes a choice, not a reflex.
Early dinners continue because you sleep better.
Simple meals stay because your digestion is happier.
And the routine holds because it feels good, not because you're forcing it.

There will still be messy days, but the difference now is that you return to your rhythm effortlessly, because it's become part of who you are.

Life after The Reset is about freedom, not from food, but from the mental clutter that used to surround it. Life is good.

Before we move on, here is a practical tip worth keeping in mind. Just like my complicated relationship with bread, my relationship with bathroom scales only works long term if I keep it casual. Scales are helpful when you are at or near your healthy weight because they give you quick feedback and help you stay aware of small changes. When you're in that stable place, you can check them regularly, even every other day, and it can be a useful way to stay on track without overthinking it.

But at the beginning of The Reset (or when returning to it), it's best to approach scales differently. Only use them after the first full week, and then only weekly. Weight fluctuates constantly, and those daily shifts can paint an inaccurate picture and trigger unnecessary concern.

The best time to weigh is first thing in the morning, after you relieve yourself and before you dress. Keep the habit consistent and do not overthink the number.

TWENTY

Social Life, Holidays, Eating Out & Alcohol: The Real World Reset

The question isn't "How do I avoid restaurants?" It's "How do I stay in my rhythm without being the bore at the dinner table?"

Many women stumble because they arrive at social events tense, hungry, or overwhelmed. When you're inflamed or overtired, you'll eat anything.

But not you, not today. You've not only survived The Reset, you've conquered it. You look and feel fabulous. You're nourished, relaxed and clear-headed.

At lunch or dinner, you naturally gravitate toward lighter, simpler meals because your body now protests when it's overwhelmed. Heavy dishes weigh you down. Rich foods leave you feeling off.

And alcohol? It becomes a conscious choice to savour with your meal, not something you gulp down before pouring another glass.

After weeks of simple, honest food that hasn't overstimulated your palate, your taste buds wake up. Your sense of smell sharpens. You're fully present, lingering over each mouthful, unhurried.

Holidays are exactly the same. You don't track a thing; you simply carry your rhythm with you.

Early dinner, when you can.
Simple lunch.

Your aunt's homemade cookies? Enjoy them, just not the whole jar in one sitting.
Plenty of walks, naturally.
Water, of course.

You don't need discipline as your regulated body does the regulating.

Restaurants become enjoyable again because you're not arriving anxious or starving. You order what you genuinely want. You stop when you're satisfied. You leave feeling good, not regretful. Dare I say it... you may have become a touch French. Ooh la la. Très chic.

Your social life stops being a threat to your goals.
It becomes an extension of your rhythm.

TWENTY-ONE

When You Slip (Because You Will): Why It Doesn't Matter

At some point, next week, next month, or six months from now, you'll have a wobble. Maybe it's stress, celebration, boredom, hormones, a bakery incident, or simply being human.

Women tend to treat these moments like failures.
"It's all ruined. I'll start again Monday."

But a slip isn't a disaster. It's just a moment. Calm your farm and return to your practice. You have the tools now.

As I said earlier and will repeat once more to cement it:
There is no wagon.
There's just life.

After The Reset you'll recognise the feeling behind the wobble: the puffiness, the restlessness, the cravings, the disconnection. Instead of spiralling, you notice it and bring yourself back.

If you add shame to a wobble, you fall into misalignment.
If you remove shame, you return to clarity.

Your body doesn't care about an occasional indulgence; it cares about being overwhelmed for days on end. Once your internal systems are balanced, they won't let you drift too far. Your appetite changes, your taste shifts, and you naturally want to protect your new energy and easy digestion. You don't need to starve or punish yourself; you simply return to your way.

Women who maintain their results aren't the ones who never slip. They're the ones who stop giving the slip too much meaning.

CHAPTER TWENTY-TWO

Your Long-Term Rhythm: The Aussie Woman Way

At some point, The Reset stops feeling like a plan and starts feeling like your normal. It arrives gradually, like the shift of a season. One day you realise you're choosing the early dinner because you sleep better. You enjoy the simple meals because they feel good. You like your routine because it grounds you.

This becomes your long-term way of living, not strict rules, but a relationship with your body that finally makes sense.

Some days feel perfect, some feel hectic, and most settle comfortably somewhere in between. This works because it respects both your physiology and your real life. Over time, the part of you that used to think about food constantly begins to quiet down.

What keeps the weight off long-term isn't restriction.
It's regulation.
Once you're regulated, everything becomes easier.

This is the moment women realise they never needed more willpower, they needed balance. And a big part of maintaining that balance is learning to live in the moment again. Not in the past, where old habits lived, and not in the future, where imagined catastrophes sit waiting. Just here, in today.

When you are present, you eat the meal in front of you, not the stress of yesterday or the pressure of tomorrow. When you are present, you move your body because it feels good, not because you are punishing it. When you are present, you notice the small changes: the ease, the lightness and the peace, instead of rushing straight past them.

Living in the now is what makes this way of eating sustainable. It turns food into a choice, not a crutch. It turns movement into a gift, not a chore. It turns your day into something you get to inhabit, not endure.

And that presence becomes its own form of nourishment.

Personally, I've set a few non-negotiables for myself. I eat at the dining table: not at my desk, not on the couch, and never with the TV on or a book in front of me. It's just the food, and the company if there is any, but no distractions. A quiet moment to enjoy a small break. Sometimes I've wanted to break this rule, but it felt important enough to keep, like a relic from slower days, something we rarely preserve in our fast-paced world. And, as with all worthwhile habits, it quietly settled in and stayed.

The long-term flow is simple:

Know yourself.
Listen to your body.
Eat calmly.
Move gently.
Rest properly.
Don't turn food into drama.

Live well and your weight follows.
It becomes a side effect, not the goal.

CHAPTER TWENTY-THREE

The Quiet Confidence You Take with You

If you've made it this far, through The Reset, embraced the rhythm, awakened to the realisations, then something bigger is unfolding than simply feeling lighter.

You've reclaimed a kind of confidence that was missing before. A quiet confidence that sinks into your bones. The quiet, deep, private knowing that you can trust yourself again.

Women spend years thinking they lack motivation, discipline, or willpower. But the truth is, you were never the problem, your system was just overwhelmed.

Once your body is regulated, you're not swimming upstream anymore. You're not negotiating with cravings or wrestling with your mood. You're not fighting exhaustion or inflammation. You're not constantly "starting again" or hunting for the next perfect plan. You're no longer stuck in that anxious, reactive state where everything feels bigger than it actually is.

When your internal world finds its balance, your external world becomes easier to navigate. This kind of confidence looks subtle from the outside. But on the inside? It changes everything.

You walk differently, not because you've lost weight, but because you're not battling yourself every day. You choose differently, not because you're being "good," but because you genuinely want to feel well. You handle social situations differently, not because you're restricting, but because you know how you want to feel the next morning. You eat differently, not out of fear, but out of clarity.

This is the freedom most women don't realise they're craving.
Not a perfect body, a quiet mind.
A body that isn't inflamed.
A stomach that isn't unpredictable.
A mood that isn't on a roller-coaster.
A life that isn't being held hostage by cravings, guilt, constipation, bloating, exhaustion, or the constant background noise of "What should I eat next?"

When I created Yeppoonie Smoothie, it solved that exact question, the what should I eat next dilemma.

And when people asked whether the smoothie powders worked for weight loss, we always said yes, providing the rest of your diet and lifestyle were in order. When people wanted more detail, we'd explain further... but as you can see from this book, the real answer is far bigger than anything I could ever fit into an email or phone call.

Hopefully this reaches the women who once asked those questions and wondered what we meant by "lifestyle in order."

When that background noise disappears, you begin to return to yourself. Not the old version, the wiser one. The woman who eats with ease, moves with intention, sleeps deeply, manages stress with a clearer perspective, chooses food that supports her and no longer gives up when she loses her way.

Confidence comes quietly in the small details of your day.
You wake with a clearer head.
You button your jeans without that familiar sinking feeling.
You say no when something doesn't feel right, and you say it without

apologising.
You put your fork down halfway through a meal because you're satisfied, not because you're trying to be good, but because you can finally hear what your body is telling you.
You catch your reflection and smile without thinking.
You laugh more.
You overthink less.
You feel slightly freer than you did last month.
You find yourself more present without needing to try so hard.

These small shifts build on one another, and together they show you that you are finding your way back to yourself in a grounded, lasting way.

And the best part?

As you learn to respect your body, these are the kinds of changes that stay with you, long after The Reset, long after the routine, long after the number on the scale stops mattering. Once you understand your body, you don't unlearn it easily. Once you feel regulated, you don't willingly return to mayhem. Once you know how to calm your appetite, soothe your stomach, support your hormones, and protect your mood, you keep doing it.

Not because you've become more disciplined,
but because you've become aligned.

This is the real gift of the Aussie Woman Reset.
Not a smaller waist, but a life that feels lighter and easier to live in.

Afterword

If you've reached the final page, you already know this wasn't really a diet book. It was a return-to-self book. A circuit-breaker. A clearing of the noise. A reminder that your body isn't broken, it's just been overwhelmed, overstimulated and completely outnumbered by modern life.

You now know that you don't need complicated plans or trendy ingredients to feel well. You don't need to turn your kitchen into a science lab or your life into a health retreat. And you certainly don't need to become more French or Japanese. You just need a steady, consistent rhythm, one that supports you rather than pressures you and actually fits the way real women live.

The most powerful part of this whole process isn't the lighter feeling or the flatter stomach (although they're a lovely bonus). It's the calm assurance that takes hold in once your body remembers how to regulate itself. It changes how you eat, how you sleep, how you think, how you respond to stress and how you carry yourself through the world.

Clarity will keep you on track. When your body feels good, you naturally make choices that keep it that way.

It was important to me that nothing here was extreme. I never wanted people to punish themselves into feeling better, that will never be sustainable. To be honest, I rarely used diet books myself, and although there are some notable exceptions, I generally find their programs either too detailed, too time-consuming, or far too restrictive. Yes, there are some limitations here: little to no alcohol, potatoes are scarce, pasta and rice are noticeably absent from the party, and yes, I temporarily broke up with bread on your behalf. But it really is short-term. And if you do have a little, it's fine. It won't undo your progress.

I wanted this reset to work, and everything here is based on what has worked for me, many times throughout my life. Yes, I stray at least once every seven years, that familiar itch, but I always find my way back. You can see now that you don't need to overhaul your entire life. You simply create space, and your body will do the rest.

Life will still be life. You'll have big days, social days, tired days, celebration days, hectic weeks, late nights out, holidays with pina coladas, cravings, moods and moments where you feel completely off your game. But the difference now is that you know how to come back to yourself. You simply return to your rhythm, the one that makes you feel centred, clear and capable.

This reset wasn't about becoming a different woman. It was about letting the real one rise to the surface, the one who isn't ruled by cravings, who isn't inflamed and overwhelmed and who doesn't let food drama consume valuable space in her life.

Aussie women have always been practical like that. We prefer things simple, manageable, and down-to-earth. And now you have a way of eating and living, that reflects that spirit....

So carry this rhythm with you. Let it be your compass, not your cage. Come back to it whenever you need to feel lighter, more at ease, or more grounded. You won't lose it now; it's part of you.

And remember, through all the seasons ahead, you're not meant to battle your body. You are meant to live in it comfortably, confidently and simply.

It took me forty-nine laps around the sun to fully realise this. It might take you less, or maybe more, but I wish you simplicity, clarity and a beautiful journey.

FAQs

Every woman has questions once The Reset begins working, especially women over 40, whose bodies do not behave the way they did in their 20s or 30s.

Here are some explanations covering:

- the psychology behind The Reset
- hormone explanations
- practical guidance
- troubleshooting
- real-life reassurance

... so you can move through your transformation without confusion, panic, or guessing.

Section 1: General Reveal FAQs

1. What if I don't feel a "Reveal Phase" in the first week?

Normal. Completely normal.

Some women feel it on Day 4.
Others Day 7.
Others Day 10 or later.

Women with:

- high stress

- poor sleep
- recent alcohol intake
- inflammation
- unpredictable eating
- hormonal fluctuations

... may take longer.

Nothing is wrong.
Your body is preparing.

Your job: stay consistent.

2. Does everyone experience Reveal Phases?

Yes, when the conditions are right.

Women over 40 absolutely have the hormonal machinery to release stored fat, fluid and inflammation... but the body needs a regulated environment to do it.

If you're:

- eating early dinners
- keeping meals simple
- cutting sugar
- staying off alcohol
- lowering stress
- sleeping better
- staying consistent

... your Reveal Phase will come.

3. How do I know a Reveal Phase is close?

Look for shifts like:

- softer belly (less firm, more "pillowy")

- lighter-feeling body
- calmer hunger
- fewer cravings
- night-time bathroom trips
- morning flatness
- improved sleep
- sudden thirst
- a sense of emotional well-being
- gentle digestive movement

If your belly suddenly feels soft instead of tight, a Reveal Phase is near.

4. What does a Reveal Phase feel like?

Women describe:

- waking up noticeably smaller
- flatter lower belly
- looser waistband
- rings suddenly fitting
- feeling "deflated" (in a good way)
- a lighter abdomen
- leggings feeling roomy

It's visible. Obvious.
Like someone turned down the inflammation dial overnight.

5. Can I speed up a Reveal Phase?

Yes, by keeping things calm:

- no alcohol
- early, simple dinners
- smoothie lunches
- eggs or protein breakfast
- cooked veggies

- herbal tea at night
- early bedtime
- low-stress days

This helps your body release instead of cling.

6. Can this be combined with an 800-calorie style plan?

Yes, if you wish but only if you are healthy and only for a short time. And never go extreme. Always check with your doctor, nutritionist, or dietitian first.

Aim for 800–1000 calories naturally through structure.

The focus of this reset is to fuel the body; not make it suffer. If you are suffering, stop.

7. Can I eat out during the 30-day reset?

Yes, easily:

- prioritise protein
- add veggies or salad
- avoid heavy creamy sauces
- avoid bread, pasta, rice
- skip dessert + alcohol combos

Restaurants are simple when you're simple.

8. What if I'm extra hungry at night?

It's usually:

- stress
- habit
- late dinners
- low protein and fibre earlier in the day

Fix it with:

- herbal tea or a caffeine-free coffee alternative such as chicory or dandelion (if you can find one that is palatable); an hour or so after dinner works well
- earlier dinner, a game-changer
- soothing evening routine, shower, bath, foot soak in magnesium salts and essential oils (even in a bucket if you have nothing else; my sad confession!)
- morning protein **and** fibre
- less screen time at night, read a book instead or talk to your family (if they are not teenagers who prefer to hibernate in their rooms; shout-out to mine)

Once hormones settle, night hunger fades.

9. Can I have coffee?

Yes, one and in the morning only.

Keep it simple (no syrup, no "milkshake in a cup").

Coffee after 2pm = cortisol spike = belly fat staying put.

10. Should I weigh myself?

On day one and then weight until about day 10.

Retention hides progress.
Scales lie.
Your clothes and waist tell the truth.

Weigh weekly (or not at all) after 10 days.

Section 2: Digestion & Bloating

1. Why am I bloated at the start?

Because your system is adjusting.

- gut bacteria shifting
- fibre increasing
- fat cells temporarily holding water
- liver clearing
- digestion re-calibrating

This is a positive sign.

The shift is coming.

2. Why am I gassy?

Your microbiome is changing. This is good.

Gas means progression, not failure.

Most women settle by Day 4–7.

3. Should I avoid raw veggies?

Yes, at first:

Cooked veg not raw veg during the early reset.

Cooked = less digestive stress and smoother Reveal Phases.

4. What if I'm constipated?

Normal in Week 1.

Do:

- warm water
- peppermint tea
- add a prune or two to your smoothies
- cooked veg
- fibre (psyllium in small amounts to smoothies/oats/yoghurt)
- light walking
- early dinners

Avoid:

- raw veg
- overeating
- stress
- late meals
- excessive almond milk if you are not used to it; try other milks. It usually resolves.

Section 3: Hormones, Menopause & The 40+ Body

1. Why do women over 40 store belly fat?

Because hormones shift:

- cortisol increases
- oestrogen fluctuates
- insulin sensitivity drops
- appetite hormones change
- sleep becomes lighter
- liver works harder

Your belly isn't "wrong."
It's responding to hormonal reality.

The Reset soothes these patterns.

2. What if I'm perimenopausal?

This structure is ideal for perimenopause.

Protein breakfast, early dinners, low sugar, predictable eating, reduced snacking, it all stabilises hormonal chaos.

3. What if I'm menopausal or post-menopausal?

You can absolutely still release fat. I did.

Once insulin settles and sleep improves, menopausal women often lose belly fat faster than younger women.

4. Why do I feel calmer on this reset?

Because your nervous system is regulated for the first time in ages:

- no sugar spikes
- no dopamine roller-coasters
- steady appetite
- lower cortisol
- peaceful evenings
- better sleep

Your body finally feels safe.

Section 4: Plateaus

1. What causes a plateau?

Usually:

- water retention
- stress
- poor sleep
- hormones shifting
- constipation
- alcohol
- fruit overload
- late dinners
- snacking

- hidden sugars

Plateaus are almost always water, not fat.

2. How do I move through a plateau?

Use the stricter 48-Hour Reset:

- eggs breakfast
- smoothie lunch
- early light dinner
- cooked veg
- no snacks
- no alcohol
- herbal tea
- early bedtime

Most women release within 48 hours.

3. How long do plateaus last?

2–7 days.
Normal, expected and harmless.

Section 5: Special Situations

1. Travelling?

Use simple rules:

one structured day, one relaxed day

or

protein and fibre breakfast daily

or

keep dinners early

You won't gain fat, just temporary water.

2. Events?

Use the **Choose One Rule**:
Alcohol **or** dessert.
Not both.

3. Bad day? Binge? Went off plan?

You didn't ruin anything.
Do not punish yourself.

Just start again at the next meal.
If in post-reset stage, you can do a quick 3-day reset to return to your equilibrium.

4. PMS?

You may feel puffy, moody, hungrier, craving everything.
Normal.

Focus on:

- protein breakfast
- cooked veg
- magnesium
- herbal tea
- early nights

You'll flatten again once hormones settle.

5. What about exercise?

Gentle is best, not intense.

Walking, yoga, Pilates, stretching are ideal.
HIIT, overtraining, long fasted workouts = cortisol spike = fat holding.

Section 6: The 12 Most Common "Why" Questions

1. Why does my lower belly stick out?

Because that's where your hormones show up first.

2. Why do I look puffy at night?

Water retention, mornings show your real shape. You will learn to love mornings again.

3. Why does appetite suddenly drop?

Your hormones have stabilised. A very good sign.

4. Why do I wake at 3am?

It's the liver's detox window. Completely temporary.

5. Why do cravings vanish?

Insulin and ghrelin settle.

6. Why do I look younger?

Inflammation drops. Sleep improves.

7. Why am I calmer?

Because you look younger, kidding.
It's really because your nervous system is no longer overloaded.

8. Why does alcohol affect me more now?

Your liver is cleaner. Sorry, not sorry.

9. Why do some days feel easier than others?

Hormones fluctuate. They always will. Such is the rhythm of life.

10. Why am I leaner after sleep?

Release happens overnight. That's why it's so important to learn to love your sleep.

11. Why do I "gain weight" after one meal?

It's water, not fat. It's gone within 24–48 hours.

12. Why does this feel so different from dieting?

Because it isn't dieting.

It's a hormone + nervous system reset, and that's why it works.

Disclaimer

The information contained in this book is intended for general informational and educational purposes only and does not constitute professional medical advice. It is not a substitute for the advice of a qualified healthcare provider. Always seek the guidance of your doctor or other qualified health professional with any questions you may have regarding a medical condition. Never disregard professional medical advice or delay in seeking it because of something you have read in this book. If you think you may have a medical emergency, call your doctor or emergency services immediately. Reliance on any information provided in this book is solely at your own risk.

This reset is designed for healthy adults and is not designed for children, pregnant or breastfeeding women, or anyone with Type 1 or insulin-dependent diabetes. If you have any medical conditions or concerns, please speak with your doctor before starting. Your health professional knows your history best. Always consult a qualified healthcare provider before making any significant dietary or lifestyle changes.

If you have any concerns, I urge you to talk to your healthcare provider. And when you do, explain it clearly:

"It's a 30–40 day reset and I'll be eating balanced meals, ideally just three times per day, with healthy snacks in between as needed while avoiding high-GI foods, alcohol, fast food, sugar, deep-fried anything and random snacking. The focus is on real food with protein, fibre, greens and staying hydrated."

APPENDIX A

The No-Nonsense Aussie Shopping List & Simple Recipes

Everything you need for the 30-Day Reset, zero fluff, zero fancy ingredients, zero fuss.

Section 1: The Essential Shopping List

This list covers everything you need for the 30-Day Reset.
You don't need all of it every week, just pick your favourites and rotate.

Protein (Choose 2–3 each week)

- Eggs
- Chicken breast or thigh (lean)
- White fish (barramundi, snapper, hake, cod)
- Lean beef
- Salmon or tinned salmon
- Tinned tuna or sardines
- Prawns
- Firm tofu or tempeh
- Cottage cheese
- Plain Greek yoghurt (unsweetened)

Veggies (Buy plenty, cooked veg are your best friend)

Cooked veg reduce bloating and help fat burn.

Choose whichever are cheapest and freshest.

- Cabbage
- Broccoli
- Leek
- Parsnip
- Brussels sprouts
- Cauliflower
- Zucchini
- Spinach or silverbeet
- Bok choy / Chinese greens
- Green beans
- Celery
- Carrots
- Capsicum
- Onion
- Garlic
- Cherry tomatoes
- Cucumbers
- Mushrooms

Fruit (Keep it minimal)

Use small amounts for smoothies or an occasional snack.

- Frozen mixed berries, organic if possible
- Bananas (freeze in small chunks)
- Apples, pears, paw paw/papaya (for snacks if needed)
- Lemons / limes

Low-GI Carbs (Optional + minimal)

You don't need these daily, they're here for backup.

- Sweet potato
- Low-GI baby potatoes

- Lentils
- Chickpeas
- Quinoa
- Rolled oats

Milks & Liquids

- Unsweetened almond milk (or milk of choice for smoothies)
- Coconut Water
- Light Coconut Milk
- Bone broth (store-bought or homemade)
- Herbal teas (peppermint, chamomile, ginger)
- Sparkling water

Flavour Add-Ons (A little goes a long way)

- Extra virgin olive/Hemp Seed/Avocado oil – choose any
- Thai red curry paste
- Balsamic vinegar
- Apple Cider Vinegar
- Soy sauce or tamari
- Garlic salt
- Onion salt
- Pepper
- Cinnamon
- Ginger (fresh or ground)
- LSA

Snacks (Low blood sugar impact)

Use sparingly and only when genuinely needed.

- Raw almonds
- Walnuts
- Raw radishes

- Boiled eggs
- Celery sticks
- Cucumber
- Greek yoghurt
- Cold-pressed juice (spinach, cucumber, ginger, ½ small carrot only)

These won't spike your blood sugar or derail your reset.

Section 2: Simple Recipes for Every Phase

Everything here is fast, simple and suits an Aussie supermarket.

Morning Calm Recipes

1. Two-Egg Protein Plate

Ingredients:

- 2 boiled eggs
- handful spinach
- 1–2 cherry tomatoes
- 2–3 tsp plain Greek yoghurt
- pepper

Method:

Assemble on a plate. Eat.
(Truly, that's it. This plate balances hormones better than any "fancy" breakfast.)

2. Basic Omelette

Ingredients:

- 2 eggs
- spinach
- onion
- mushrooms (optional)

- tomato (optional)
- capsicum (optional)

Method:

Whisk eggs → pan → add veg → cook gently → fold.
Zero drama, maximum stability.

3. Greek Yoghurt Mini Bowl

For mornings when you're not very hungry or add to overnight oats if you are.

- ½ cup Greek yoghurt
- pinch cinnamon
- ¼ cup berries
- 1 tsp chia seeds (optional)

Midday Nourish Recipes

1. Yeppoonie-Style Smoothie

Ingredients:

- 250-300 ml unsweetened almond milk
- ⅓ cup frozen berries + banana (combined)
- 1 scoop protein powder or Yeppoonie blend
- 1 big spoon plain Greek yoghurt

Blend. Sip. Done.
Gut-friendly, low-GI, calming.

2. Chicken & Veg Bowl

Ingredients:

- Approx 100 g cooked chicken
- steamed broccoli
- cabbage
- zucchini

- squeeze lemon
- pepper

Method:

Warm everything → season → eat.
Takes 5 minutes if meal-prepped.

3. Tuna Crunch Salad

Ingredients:

- 1 tin tuna
- cucumber
- tomato
- lettuce
- onion
- spinach
- tiny drizzle olive oil
- lemon or balsamic

Fresh, light, anti-inflammatory.

4. Broth Bowl

Ingredients:

- bone broth
- greens (bok choy, spinach)
- chicken or boiled egg

Heat broth → drop in protein + greens → 3 minutes → done.

Early Evening Reset Recipes

1. Lemon Chicken & Greens

Ingredients:

- 100 g chicken

- broccoli + cabbage (cooked)
- lemon
- pepper

Method:

Pan-sear chicken lightly → steam veg → plate with lemon.

2. Simple Fish Bowl

Ingredients:

- white fish fillet
- zucchini
- bok choy
- ginger
- lime

Pan-sear fish → wilt greens → squeeze lime.

3. Protein + Soup Combo

Ingredients:

- bone broth
- any cooked veg
- shredded chicken

Heat and serve for a gentle, digestion-friendly dinner.

Section 3, Low-Impact Snacks (Only When Necessary)

Use sparingly and only when genuinely hungry, not bored, stressed or procrastinating.

- a small handful of raw almonds
- 1 boiled egg
- a radish or two (crunchy and perfect)

- 2–3 spoons Greek yoghurt
- 1 piece of fruit (apple, pear or berries)
- cold-pressed green juice (spinach, cucumber, ginger, ½ small carrot only)

These options will not spike blood sugar or ruin progress.

Section 4: 10-Minute Dinners (For Exhausted Days)

Choose **any** of these on nights you're over it:

1. **Eggs + Greens**
   2–3 eggs scrambled or boiled + any cooked vegetables.
2. **Tuna Plate**
   Tin tuna + cucumber + tomato + lettuce + drizzle olive oil and balsamic
3. **Chicken Soup Bowl**
   Bone broth + leftover chicken + bok choi + leek + vegetables on hand
4. **Stir-Together Veg Bowl**
   Sauté zucchini + cabbage + capsicum + onion + add protein.
5. **Yoghurt Mini Dinner (only when appetite is tiny)**
   Greek yoghurt + cinnamon + berries.

Seven Smoothies You Can Make If You Don't Have Yeppoonie Smoothie

These are:

- low GI
- high fibre
- high protein

They will keep you full and energised.

1. **Berry Protein Fibre Smoothie**
    - 1 cup mixed berries
    - 1 scoop protein powder
    - 1 tbsp chia seeds
    - ½ cup Greek yoghurt
    - water or almond milk
2. **Coconut Vanilla Oat Fibre Smoothie**
    - ½ scoop protein powder
    - ¼ cup oats
    - 1 tbsp psyllium husk or chia seeds
    - ½ banana
    - coconut water and almond milk mix (50/50)
3. **Green Gut-Health Protein Smoothie**
    - 1 scoop protein powder
    - 1 cup spinach
    - ½ cucumber
    - ¼ avocado
    - 1 tbsp ground flaxseed
    - water or almond milk
4. **Apple Pie Protein Smoothie**
    - 1 small green apple (chopped or lightly steam then cool if your blender isn't very powerful)
    - 1 scoop vanilla protein
    - 1 tbsp oats
    - 1 tsp cinnamon
    - water or almond milk
5. **Blueberry Almond Smoothie**
    - 1 cup blueberries
    - 1 scoop protein powder

- 1 tbsp ground almonds or almond butter
- 1 teaspoon chia seeds
- almond milk

6. **Carrot Cake Protein Smoothie**
   - 1 small carrot (chopped or lightly steam then cool if your blender isn't very powerful)
   - ½ banana or 1–2 dates (optional)
   - 1 scoop protein
   - 1 tbsp ground flaxseed
   - cinnamon + ginger
   - almond milk

7. **Chocolate Fibre Protein Shake**
   - 1 scoop chocolate protein
   - 2 tsp psyllium husk
   - 1 tsp chia or flax
   - 1 tsp cacao powder (optional)
   - water or almond milk

APPENDIX B

Useful Websites & Resources

Nutrition & Healthy Eating

- **Glycaemic Index Foundation (Australia)**
  www.gisymbol.com
  Evidence-based information on GI, GL and low-GI foods.

- **Nutrition Australia**
  www.nutritionaustralia.org
  General nutrition guidance, healthy eating tips and current dietary recommendations.

- **The Gut Health Foundation**
  www.guthealth.org
  Resources on digestion, microbiome support and gut-friendly eating.

Hormones, Women's Health & Menopause

- **Jean Hailes for Women's Health**
  www.jeanhailes.org.au
  Australia's leading women's health resource, hormones, menopause, perimenopause and healthy ageing.

- **Australasian Menopause Society**
  www.menopause.org.au
  Reliable information on midlife health, hormone therapy and symptom management.

Mental Wellbeing & Stress Support

- **Beyond Blue**
  www.beyondblue.org.au
  Clear, practical support for stress, anxiety and mental wellbeing.

- **Black Dog Institute**
  www.blackdoginstitute.org.au
  Evidence-based resources on mood, resilience and emotional health.

Movement & Lifestyle

- **Physical Activity Guidelines – Australia**
  www.health.gov.au/health-topics/physical-activity
  Up-to-date guidelines for movement, exercise and healthy ageing.

- **Pilates Alliance Australasia**
  www.pilates.org.au
  Information on Pilates instructors, classes and benefits.

Books

- **4 Ingredients *More Diabetes* by Kim McCosker**
  www.4ingredients.com.au
  Super simple and healthy recipes that pair beautifully with post-reset eating for diabetics. Reviewed by Diabetes Victoria.

- **4 Ingredients *Healthy Diet* by Kim McCosker**
  www.4ingredients.com.au
  Super simple and healthy recipes that pair beautifully with post-reset eating for everyone.

APPENDIX C

Calories & Kilojoules per 100 g and per 50 g

PROTEINS

Food	kcal (100 g)	kJ (100 g)	kcal (50 g)	kJ (50 g)
Eggs (whole)	143	598	72	299
Chicken breast (lean)	165	690	82	345
Chicken thigh (lean)	209	874	104	437
White fish (barramundi/snapper/hake/cod)	90	377	45	188
Lean beef	250	1050	125	525
Salmon (fresh)	206	862	103	431
Salmon (tinned, springwater)	136	570	68	285
Tuna (tinned, springwater)	116	485	58	242
Sardines (tinned)	208	870	104	435
Prawns	99	414	50	207
Tofu (firm)	144	603	72	302
Tempeh	193	808	96	404

Cottage cheese (low-fat)	98	410	49	205
Greek yoghurt (unsweetened)	59	246	30	123

VEGETABLES

Food	kcal (100 g)	kJ (100 g)	kcal (50 g)	kJ (50 g)
Cabbage	25	105	12	52
Broccoli	34	142	17	71
Leek	61	255	30	128
Parsnip	75	314	38	157
Brussels sprouts	43	180	22	90
Cauliflower	25	105	12	52
Zucchini	17	71	8	36
Spinach	23	96	12	48
Silverbeet / Chard	19	79	10	40
Bok choy	13	54	6	27
Green beans	31	130	16	65
Celery	16	67	8	34
Carrots	41	172	20	86
Capsicum	31	130	16	65

Onion	40	167	20	84
Garlic	149	623	74	312
Cherry tomatoes	18	75	9	38
Cucumbers	15	63	8	32
Mushrooms	22	92	11	46

FRUIT

Food	**kcal (100 g)**	**kJ (100 g)**	**kcal (50 g)**	**kJ (50 g)**
Mixed berries (frozen)	50	209	25	104
Bananas	89	371	44	186
Apples	52	218	26	109
Pears	57	239	28	120
Pawpaw / Papaya	43	180	22	90
Lemons / Limes	29	121	14	60

LOW-GI CARBS

Food	**kcal (100 g)**	**kJ (100 g)**	**kcal (50 g)**	**kJ (50 g)**
Sweet potato	86	360	43	180

Baby potatoes (low-GI)	87	365	44	182
Lentils (cooked)	116	485	58	242
Chickpeas (cooked)	164	686	82	343
Quinoa (cooked)	120	502	60	251
Rolled oats (dry)	389	1630	194	815

MILKS & LIQUIDS

Food	**kcal (100 g)**	**kJ (100 g)**	**kcal (50 g)**	**kJ (50 g)**
Almond milk (unsweetened)	15	63	8	32
Coconut water	19	80	10	40
Light coconut milk	136	568	68	284
Bone broth	40	167	20	84
Herbal tea	0	0	0	0
Sparkling water	0	0	0	0

FLAVOUR ADD-ONS & OILS

Food	kcal (100 g)	kJ (100 g)	kcal (50 g)	kJ (50 g)
Extra virgin olive oil	884	3699	442	1850
Avocado oil	884	3699	442	1850
Hemp seed oil	884	3699	442	1850
Apple Cider Vinegar	21	88	10.5	44
Thai red curry paste	142	594	71	297
Balsamic vinegar	88	368	44	184
Soy sauce	53	222	26	111
Tamari	60	251	30	126
Pepper	251	1050	126	525
Cinnamon	247	1034	124	517
Ginger (fresh)	80	335	40	168
Ginger (ground)	335	1400	168	700
LSA	536	2240	268	1120

SNACKS

Food	kcal (100 g)	kJ (100 g)	kcal (50 g)	kJ (50 g)
Raw almonds	579	2423	290	1212
Radishes	16	67	8	34
Boiled egg	155	648	78	324
Celery sticks	16	67	8	34
Cucumber slices	15	63	8	32
Greek yoghurt (unsweetened)	59	246	30	123
Cold-pressed green juice	40	167	20	84
Walnuts	654	2730	327	1365

APPENDIX D

Shopping List Guide (Printable)

A useful guide, you don't need to buy everything at once. Tick what suits your week.

A useful guide, you don't need to buy everything at once. Tick what suits your week.

Proteins:

- ☐ Eggs
- ☐ Chicken
- ☐ White fish
- ☐ Salmon/tuna (tinned)
- ☐ Prawns
- ☐ Salmon
- ☐ Beef (lean mince or steak)
- ☐ Tofu/tempeh
- ☐ Cottage cheese
- ☐ Greek yoghurt

Veggies:

- ☐ Cabbage
- ☐ Broccoli
- ☐ Cauliflower
- ☐ Zucchini
- ☐ Spinach
- ☐ Bok choy

- ☐ Tomatoes
- ☐ Cucumbers
- ☐ Mushrooms
- ☐ Onions
- ☐ Garlic
- ☐ Carrots
- ☐ Celery
- ☐ Brussels sprouts
- ☐ Leek

Fruit:

- ☐ Berries – fresh and frozen (for smoothies)
- ☐ Bananas
- ☐ Apples/pears
- ☐ Lemons/limes
- ☐ Pawpaw

Liquids:

- ☐ Almond milk unsweetened (Pure Harvest from Supermarkets is great)
- ☐ Bone broth (Nutra Organics from health food stores is my go-to)
- ☐ Lite coconut milk
- ☐ Herbal teas

Pantry Basics / Pantry Staples

- ☐ Extra Virgin Olive/Hemp Seed/Avocado (any preferred)
- ☐ Balsamic vinegar
- ☐ Apple cider vinegar
- ☐ Soy sauce
- ☐ Chili paste
- ☐ Chili flakes
- ☐ Sea salt

- ☐ Pepper
- ☐ Cinnamon
- ☐ Psyllium
- ☐ Spices
- ☐ Raw oats
- ☐ Herbal tea
- ☐ Nutritional yeast
- ☐ LSA

Optional:

- ☐ Almonds
- ☐ Radishes
- ☐ Kefir (milk or water if you can find it)
- ☐ Ginger
- ☐ Kimchi
- ☐ Chia seeds
- ☐ Pumpkin seeds
- ☐ Hemp seeds
- ☐ Fresh ginger
- ☐ Real sourdough or dense rye bread sliced thin

Made in the USA
Monee, IL
04 November 2026

67378036R00089